TRANSGENIC CROPS - EMERGING TRENDS AND FUTURE PERSPECTIVES

Edited by **Muhammad Sarwar Khan**
and **Kauser Abdulla Malik**

Transgenic Crops - Emerging Trends and Future Perspectives
http://dx.doi.org/10.5772/intechopen.73723
Edited by Muhammad Sarwar Khan and Kauser Abdulla Malik

Contributors

Phetole Mangena, Ian Dubery, Lerato Matsaunyane, Mohammad Sayyar Khan, Mudassar Nawaz Khan, Mousa Mousavi, Mohsen Brajeh, Jorge Ricaño-Rodríguez, Jorge Suárez-Medellin, Eliezer Cocoletzi Vásquez, José María Ramos-Prado, Enrique Hipólito-Romero1, Ghulam Mustafa, Muhammad Sarwar Khan, Faiz Ahmad, Kauser Malik

First published in London, United Kingdom, 2019 by IntechOpen
IntechOpen is the global imprint of INTECHOPEN LIMITED, registered in England and Wales, registration number: 11086078, The Shard, 25th floor, 32 London Bridge Street
London, SE19SG – United Kingdom
Printed in Croatia

British Library Cataloguing-in-Publication Data
A catalogue record for this book is available from the British Library

Additional hard and PDF copies can be obtained from orders@intechopen.com

Transgenic Crops - Emerging Trends and Future Perspectives , Edited by Muhammad Sarwar Khan and Kauser Abdulla Malik
p. cm.
Print ISBN 978-1-83962-492-6
Online ISBN 978-1-83962-493-3
eBook (PDF) ISBN 978-1-83962-494-0

For EU product safety concerns:
IN TECH d.o.o., Prolaz Marije Krucifikse Kozulić 3, 51000 Rijeka, Croatia,
info@intechopen.com or visit our website at intechopen.com.

Meet the editors

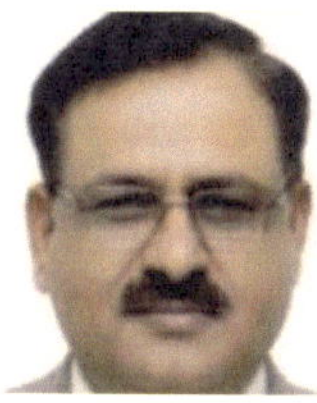

Muhammad Sarwar Khan is currently serving as Professor and Director at the Center of Agricultural Biochemistry and Biotechnology (CABB), University of Agriculture, Faisalabad, Pakistan. He has earned his Ph.D. from the University of Cambridge, UK. Afterward, he was awarded the Rockefeller foundation fellowship under the Rice Biotechnology Program for Developing Countries to carry out research at the Waksman Institute of Microbiology, Rutgers, USA. His first of its kind research was published in Nature Biotechnology. Dr. Khan has served as the founding group leader of Chloroplast Transformation and Biopharming, and as the head of Biotech Interdisciplinary Division at NIBGE. Dr. Khan has supervised more than 100 Ph.D., M-Phil students, and researchers.
He has published 50 articles in high impact journals, including Nature, and he is the author of several book chapters and books. Dr. Khan has developed transgenic sugarcane, resistant to top borers and tolerant to a herbicide, which was approved by the National Biosafety Committee (NBC) for field trials in 2006–2007. This was the first proposal of endogenously developed transgenic crops, approved by the NBC in Pakistan. Dr. Khan has also pioneered plastid transformation in rice and sugarcane, recalcitrant plant species. He has also knocked out a number of genes from the chloroplast genome of higher plants. His current research interests include the development of edible-marker-carrying transgenics, cost-effective therapeutics and edible vaccines for animals. Dr. Khan has received prestigious national and international awards and is on the Editorial Boards of international scientific journals.

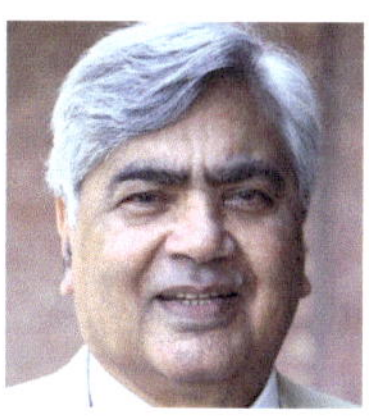

Kauser Abdulla Malik, currently working as Professor and Dean of Postgraduate Studies at Forman Christian College (a Chartered University), Lahore, received his PhD in Microbiology from the University of Aston, UK. He is an Alexander von Humboldt Fellow and worked at the Institute of Soil Biochemistry in Braunschweig, Germany. In Pakistan he worked at the Nuclear Institute for Agriculture and Biology and later as founder Director of the National Institute for Biotechnology and Genetic Engineering at Faisalabad. Dr. Malik has been the Chairman of the Pakistan Agriculture Research Council, a member of the Biosciences at Pakistan Atomic Energy Commission, and a member of the Food and Agri of Planning Commission of Pakistan. He has been a Higher Education Commission Distinguished National Professor since 2005. He was awarded the ISESCO Prize in Biology in 1997. Dr. Malik's areas of research are in molecular biology of plant–microbe interactions and metagenomics and transgenics for biofortification and biopharmaceuticals with over 250 peer-reviewed publications, seven patents, five edited books, and several book chapters. He has been awarded three civil awards for his contributions to science by the presidents of Pakistan. He is an elected Fellow of the Pakistan Academy of Sciences and the World Academy of Sciences.

Contents

Preface

Transgenic crops are referred to as genetically engineered crops. Traits, otherwise impossible to introduce by conventional breeding techniques, are tailored using genetic manipulation and transformation approaches. While developing transgenics, biotechnologists have paid much attention to improving crops to withstand the devastating effects of biotic and abiotic stresses, including insects, pathogens, weeds, salinity, and drought. Advancement in recombinant technology augurs well in the development of transgenics expressing nutraceuticals, pharmaceuticals, and antigenic proteins (vaccines) for humans and livestock. Henceforth, this book discusses the state-of-the-art advances in this rapidly developing area of transgenic technology, a technology for the food and health security of mainly poor people in developing countries where populations and urbanization are rapidly increasing.

Transgenic Crops - Emerging Trends and Future Perspectives consists of seven chapters. The flow of chapters in the book is strategically organized to allow for easy reading. It begins with Chapter 1 in which Drs. Muhammad Sarwar Khan and Kauser Abdulla Malik demonstrate comprehensively how novel molecular biology approaches could be used to develop transgenic crops for agronomic and medicinal traits. In Chapter 2, Dr. Mangena explains the factors affecting efficient regeneration of transgenic plants developed through an *Agrobacterium*-mediated method of genome engineering. Dr. Ricaño-Rodríguez and his team in Chapter 3 propose the use of CRISPR/Cas9 technology that has allowed the generation of diverse molecular methodologies to constitute significant advances in the genome edition and its subsequent exploitation for agricultural and medicinal purposes. In Chapter 4, Dr. Khan and his team discuss the emerging trends in chloroplast biotechnology, and highlight the use of the technology in the sustainable production of food and expensive molecules. Drs. Muhammad Sayyar Khan and Mudassar Nawaz Khan suggest in Chapter 5 how developments in -omics approaches have revolutionized the biotechnology field for crop improvement against drought and salinity stresses. Drs. Mousavi and Fard very comprehensively highlight genetic improvement of commercially important tropical and subtropical fruit trees, including banana, date palm, citrus, mango, olive, and pineapple in Chapter 6. Drs. Matsaunyane and Dubery discuss the pros and cons of developing transgenic plants in Chapter 7, and suggest that the unattended effects of gene insertions into the genomes be brought about while analyzing the transgenic plants for differential gene expression profiling, keeping in view safety assessment guidelines and requirements.

Muhammad Sarwar Khan, PhD
Professor and Director
Center of Agricultural Biochemistry and Biotechnology
University of Agriculture, Faisalabad, Pakistan

Kauser Abdulla Malik, PhD
Professor and Dean
Forman Christian College (A Chartered University), Lahore, Pakistan

Chapter 1

Introductory Chapter: Transgenics—Crops Tailored for Novel Traits

Muhammad Sarwar Khan and Kauser Abdulla Malik

Additional information is available at the end of the chapter

http://dx.doi.org/10.5772/intechopen.81372

1. Introduction

Transgenic crops are referred to as the genetically engineered crops. Traits, otherwise impossible to introduce by conventional approaches, are tailored using genetic manipulations and transformation approaches. Among traits is the introduction of agronomic, pathological, entomological, nutritional, therapeutic-, and vaccine-related characters in plants. The chapter covers state-of-the-art advancements in this rapidly developing area of transgenic technology and the technology for the food and health security mainly of poor populace in the developing countries.

This era has seen an explosive growth in population and urbanization, leading to an immense loss of agricultural land; therefore, the food security, especially which of poor populace, is of foremost importance. According to an estimate, this requires approximately 70% increment in food production by 2050. Since the 1990s, the introduction of insect resistance and herbicide tolerance into transgenic crops has increased the yield tremendously, benefiting farmers worldwide. Though production is increased by addressing problems of yield losses using transgenic technology, malnutrition is still one of the biggest challenges, demanding fortification of grains. Since nutrition is one of the main factors in maintaining a healthy lifestyle and meeting requirements of food security, several national nutrition surveys conducted in various countries have provided an avenue for governments to assess malnutrition problems across populations. Micronutrient deficiencies have been termed as the cause of "hidden hunger." Iron-fortified products are the prime examples of it. Pyramiding genes that encode provitamin A, transgenically or naturally, in crops like rice [1], potatoes [2], and maize [3, 4] have made these crops a rich source of provitamin A. In addition to adding nutritional elements in crops, the transgenic technology has led the scientists to tailor medicinal traits, for example, therapeutic [5, 6] and antigen proteins [7].

Transgenic crops are developed in routine to express agricultural and medicinal traits, but it is very important to discuss the technologies used to develop them. Nuclear transformation is more successful in tailoring agricultural traits in crops (**Figure 1**), though it remained unfruitful in few genotypes like upland cotton in the Indo-Pak subcontinent, the reason being these genotypes are recalcitrant to regeneration from single cell, despite several crosses were made between genotypes to improve the regeneration potential, while chloroplast transformation is distinctly effective to tailor medicinal traits (**Figure 2**) [5, 6], the reason being nutraceutical, pharmaceutical, and antigenic proteins are required to be accumulated in exceptionally high amounts with bona fide structures. Chloroplasts are polyploid at organellar and genome levels and provide natural gene containment [8]; hence, they are preferred

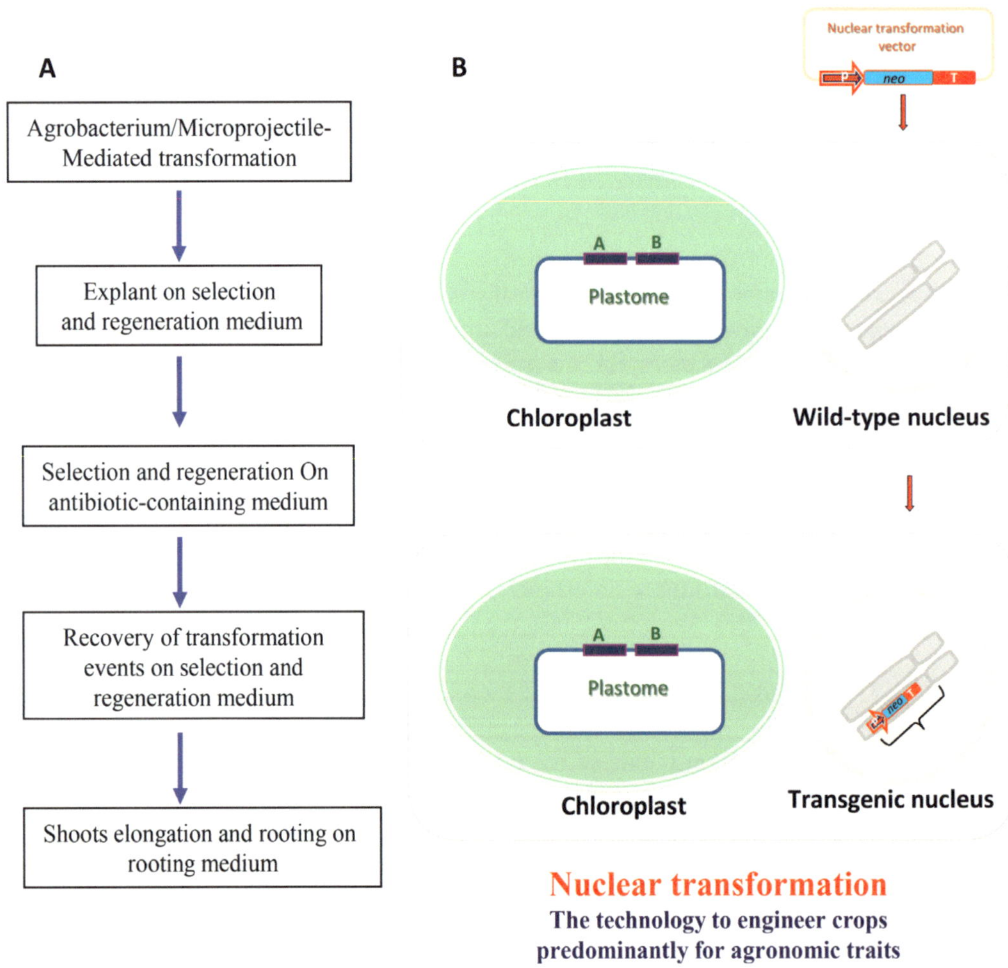

Figure 1. Transgenics predominantly for agronomic traits. Panel A explains the transformation steps involved in the development of transgenics. Panel B shows integration of transgene into the nuclear genome of crops via *Agrobacterium*-mediated or ballistic transformation approaches where transformation vector is either bombarded or cloned between left and right borders of a plasmid vector and multiplication using suitable *Agrobacterium* strain.

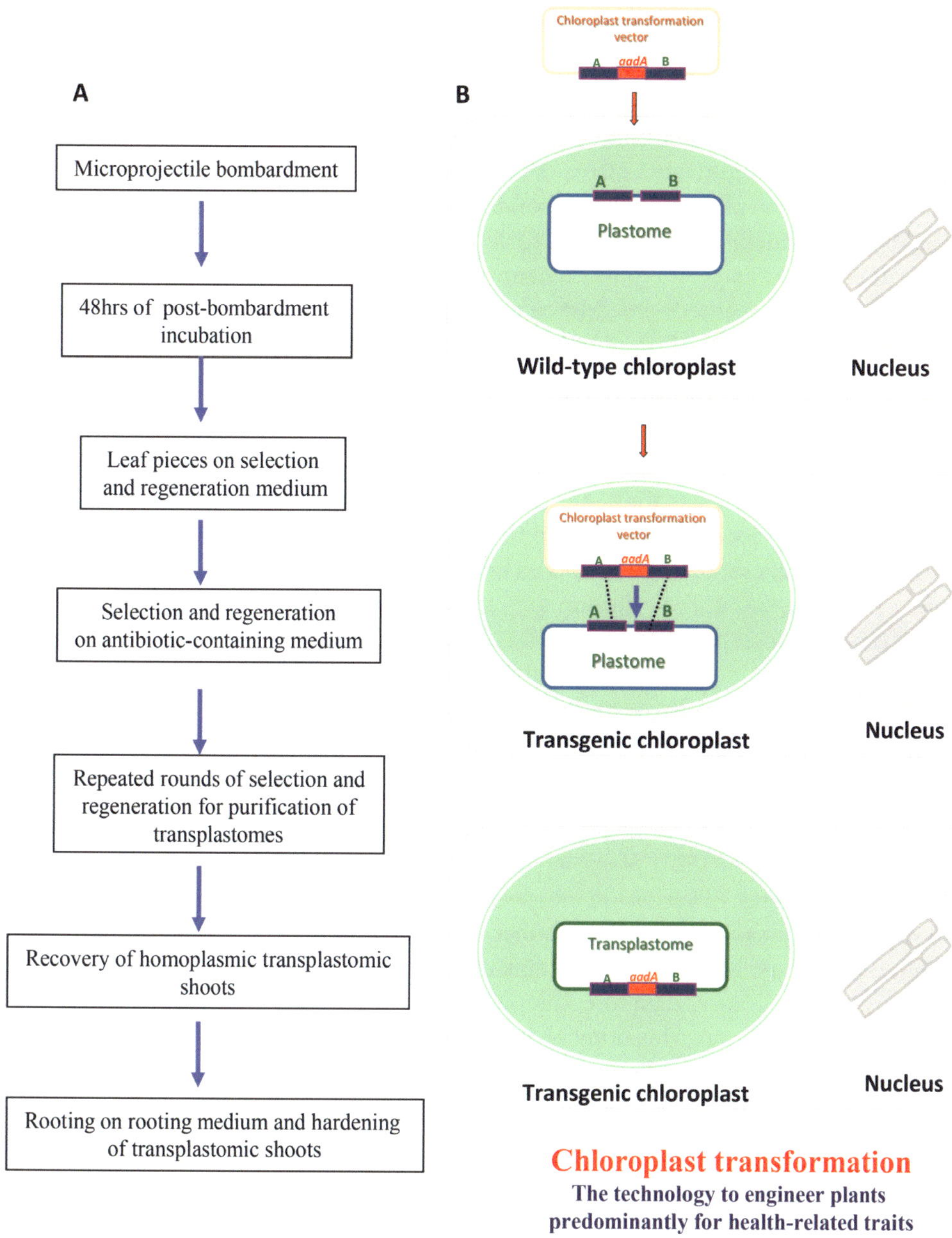

Figure 2. Transgenics predominantly for health-related traits. Panel A explains main steps involved in the development of transgenic chloroplasts to express transgenes that encode novel proteins to be used as nutraceuticals, therapeutics or vaccines. Panel B explains how a transgene from a transformation vector is integrated into the plastome via homologous recombination events to accumulate proteins to high levels with *bona fide* structures.

to express health-related traits rather agricultural. Plastid transformation though is achieved in wheat [9], rice [10], and sugarcane, but it is reproducible only in rice [11], yet transgenic plants remain heteroplasmic.

2. Developing transgenics: state-of-the-art strategies

A plant cell is blessed with three major organelles with their own genomes, namely, nucleus, chloroplast, and mitochondria. Of these three, two genomes are routinely manipulated to incorporate new traits in cultivated plants. There are a number of approaches to transfer and introduce genes into the plant genome, depending upon the choice of explant to be used in transformation experiments, for example, *Agrobacterium*-mediated gene transfer, gene gun, agro-infiltration, sonication, and polyethylene glycol treatment. Of these, *Agrobacterium*-mediated and gene gun methods are most commonly used approaches to develop transgenic plants. For nuclear transformation, *Agrobacterium* method is more successful than particle bombardment as a more number of transformed shoots can be recovered from the same number of explant.

Genetic transformation process involves a number of steps, including selection of a gene that confers resistance to a particular antibiotic for selection and screening purposes, isolation of a trait-encoding gene, choice of promoters and terminating sequences to control the expression of the gene or genes, choice of explant, and an artificial medium to support explant to regenerate into a complete shoot. For selection and screening, usually two types of markers are used: (1) selectable marker and (2) visual marker [10, 12–14]. Selectable marker could be lethal or nonlethal in nature. Nuclear genome transformation is carried out using lethal markers. Regenerated shoots are normally hemi- or heterozygous and need either further purification of transgenome using selection medium or through selfing depending upon the crop used.

The second genome is the chloroplast genome, the plastome that has been modified in a number of plant species, including model, crop, and tree plants. Plastome is a double-stranded DNA molecule of 152 (*Cinnamomum campohra*) – 218 kb (*Pelargonium*) size [15, 16]. Approximately, 120 genes in various plant species are encoded by the plastome [17]. It looks like that most of the ancestral genes have either been lost during evolution or transferred to the nucleus. A mature mesophyll cell contains up to 100 chloroplasts, and each chloroplast contains 100 plastome copies; therefore, the ploidy number of plastome per cell reaches up to 10,000 copies. Furthermore, this number is doubled for genes that are located in inverted repeat regions of the plastome [17].

When transforming a chloroplast, a universal antibiotic cannot be used given that different plants have variable sensitivity to selective agents; therefore, recovery of the transplastomic shoots is dependent on two things: (1) choice of the selective agent to be used and (2) the concentration of the selective agent that allows regeneration and development of shoots from the transformed cells while killing the non-transformed cells. For example, spectinomycin is used to select transformed cells on selection medium from tobacco, lettuce, tomato, potato, cabbage, oil rape seed, and carrot. However, several monocots, including rice and sugarcane, are naturally resistant to spectinomycin; therefore, streptomycin-containing medium was used for carrying out selection for transplastomic lines.

Initially, only few copies of the plastid genome are transformed and maintained under continuous selection pressure. However, stable lines with uniformly transformed genome copies are recovered on selection medium through a repeated cycle of regeneration [6]. During the period, the wild-type and the transgenic plastids and their genomes gradually sort out;

thereby, chimeric sectors, carrying wild-type or transgenic plastids, appear in leaves of regenerated shoots. Due to phenotypic masking by the transformed cells, both transgenic and wild-type cells in a chimeric shoot look green in color [6], indicating that antibiotic resistance is not cell autonomous. However, both wild-type and transformed sectors are identifiable using green fluorescent protein (GFP). This visual marker allows visual detection of the fluorescing transproteins because they produce green fluorescence upon illumination with blue or ultraviolet (UV) light [18, 6].

3. Transgenics for agricultural traits

3.1. Transgenics to improve crop production

Plants on earth synthesize their food by themselves, owing to harbor solar energy conversion and several other chemical reactions in their cells. One of the reactions carried out in plants is carbon fixation during a process, namely, photosynthesis. During photosynthesis Rubisco catalyzes the inefficient carbon fixation, reviewed extensively elsewhere [19, 20]. This raises a question why carbon fixation during photosynthesis is rate limiting. Major reasons are as follows: first, Rubisco's rate of catalysis is much low, and, second, it has to compete with a nonproductive reaction, oxygenation [21], depending upon the relative concentration of carbon dioxide and oxygen, as well as on temperature. Carboxylation results in CO_2 fixation. Therefore, plant growth and yield can be improved by two ways: (1) by increasing photosynthesis and (2) by reducing photorespiration.

A number of examples are available in the literature, reporting different versions of Rubisco that would improve photosynthesis [22], but considerable success has not been achieved yet. Introducing C_4 pathway in C_3 plants appears to be more promising, but due to the leakage of gases, the advantages of concentrating carbon dioxide in the chloroplasts of C_3 plants are objectionable [23]. Glycolate catabolic pathway was introduced in chloroplasts for alleviation of photorespiratory losses in *Arabidopsis thaliana*. Photosynthesis is markedly increased in this engineered pathway, thereby widening the applicability of the technique to cereals, for example, wheat and rice, described in detail elsewhere [24].

Developing chlorophyll in the dark, and chloroplasts that are competent for photosynthesis upon exposure to light, is another promising technique that can be implied to improve the photosynthesis in plants [25, 26]. In a study, *chlB* gene from *Pinus thunbergii* was introduced into the plastome of *Nicotiana tabacum* [27]. Transgenic plants when shifted to light from dark in early development of chlorophyll pigments were observed in leaves of transgenic compared to wild-type plants. This helps us to understand the molecular biology of transgenic angiosperms. Another effort is underway to introduce C_4 pathway in rice, a C_3 plant [28], using various techniques.

3.2. Transgenics for weed management

Weeds compete with crops for food, thereby lowering the crop yield and affecting farmers. There are two types of herbicides, (1) selective in nature and (2) used before and after emergence of plants from seeds, and are specific to leaf morphology.

A pioneering concept to engineer a crop for herbicide tolerance was developed in the 1980s [29] when it was observed that few herbicides kill plants by blocking photosynthetic electron transport. For example, triazine herbicides bind to a photosystem-II protein (D1) in the chloroplasts that appeared to be the first molecular target to develop a commercial herbicide [30]. However, tolerance to herbicides in transgenic plants is considered the best approach in weed control in crops. Glyphosate is a nonselective broad-spectrum herbicide that kills narrow-leaf grasses and broad-leaf weeds. Glyphosate competitively inhibits 5-enol-pyruvyl shikimate-3-phosphate synthase (EPSP) in the amino acid biosynthetic pathway. This proves to be a standard strategy to overcome the problem of herbicide selectivity. Yet, this strategy raises the concern of gene transfer to other plants or weeds.

An antibiotic bialaphos inhibits glutamine synthetase (GS) upon removal of alanine residues in the nitrogen assimilation pathway; resultantly, accumulation of toxic levels of ammonia in both bacteria and plant cells occurs. This antibiotic was used as an herbicide that appeared to be nonselective in nature. In two different studies, transgenic tobacco plants exhibited field-level tolerance to phosphinothricin (PPT) when bar was expressing from chloroplast genome [31, 32]. Further, development of glufosinate-resistant traits has been reported worldwide in corn, soybean, and cotton until now. The trait has also been developed by Khan and his team in sugarcane, and the transgenic plants were tolerant to BASTA [33]. The extensive and continuous use of a single herbicide should be avoided to exclude the possibilities of resistance development in plants, and precautionary measures should be taken to safeguard human health.

3.3. Transgenics for insect resistance

Engineering plant genomes for useful traits leads toward sustainable agriculture. Among useful traits, resistance against insects is developed by using Cry proteins from *Bacillus thuringiensis* (*Bt*). *Bacillus thuringiensis* is a soilborne bacterium, having crystal (Cry) proteins in the cytoplasm of the cells at sporulating stage. These proteins are toxic to some chewing and sucking insects.

Genes encoding Cry proteins have been expressed in a number of crops worldwide to control major pests. This has reduced the pesticide usage and has lowered the production costs of crops. First, transgenic crops developed were corn and cotton that expressed *cry1Ab* and *cry1Ac* genes, respectively [34]. Afterward, other crops including soybean, maize, cotton, canola, squash, papaya, tomato, sugar beet, and sugarcane were transformed using *Bt* genes to control insects. Almost all global biotech crop area is because of soybean, corn, cotton, and canola crops [35]. Since the first commercial cultivation of GM crops in 1996, farmers (16.7 million) from 29 countries cultivated 160 million hectares of biotech crops in 2011. Out of this number, about 90% were small and resource poor farmers belonging to developing countries. The United States and Brazil were major producers who adopted GM crops.

In Pakistan, first indigenously developed transgenic crop was sugarcane, carrying *cry1Ab* gene that was approved by the Technical Advisory and National Biosafety Committees after the approval of biosafety rules and guidelines in 2005. Developed sugarcane plants carry

Bt toxin only in green tops with no residues in the juice [36]. Lately, a different version of the *cry1Ab* gene was again used to develop transgenic sugarcane, and similar results were obtained.

3.4. Transgenics for pathogen resistance

Plant pathogens are damaging plants and causing yield losses exceptionally; it is therefore highly desirable to develop transgenics that would be resistant to pathogenic bacteria and fungi. There are a number of examples available in literature where pathogens have been targeted to control diseases in plants. Arrieta and colleagues in 1996 reported co-expression of genes encoding glucanase- and thaumitin-like proteins, and a low level of fungal infection was observed [37]. In other studies when snakin-1 gene was overexpressed transgenically, an enhanced resistance to *Rhizoctonia solani* and *Erwinia carotovora* was observed. Similarly, chitinase gene from *Streptomyces griseus* showed resistance against *Alternaria solani*, while expression of mycoparasitic chitinase and glucanase enzymes developed improved resistance to *Rhizoctonia solani*. Five novel thionin genes were isolated from plants belonging to the *Brassicaceae* family, and when expressed transgenically in potato, a high-degree resistance to gray mold (*Botrytis cinerea*) was observed [38]. Literature review suggests that broad-spectrum resistance could be attained in valuable plant species through transgenic technology. Mycoparasites can be controlled using glucanases, chitinases, proteases, cellulases, kinases, and certain antibiotics.

Amphipathic peptides such as magainin are known to control microbe infections; Daniell and his colleagues expressed MSI-99 in chloroplasts of tobacco and reported a varied degree resistance to microbes [39] with no changes in growth and development of the transgenic plants compared to wild-type plants. But using such genes in crops warrants extensive biosafety studies.

4. Transgenics for medicinal traits

4.1. Transgenics for nutraceuticals

One of the items on the wish list of biotechnologists is to engineer genomes of plants to tailor high-value traits other than agronomic, pathological, and entomological in nature. Among high-value traits are the introduction of nutrition and related characters. "Nutraceuticals" is a portmanteau of "nutrition" and "pharmaceuticals"; hence, the word implies that nutraceuticals are products regulated as medicine, food ingredients, and dietary supplements. These products not only provide protection against various diseases caused due to the deficiency of the nutrients but also have physiological benefits. Traditionally, nutraceuticals have been employed in the form of medicinal plants, etc., but in this modern era, nutraceuticals are being used in a variety of perspectives, such as nutrition and medicine. Iron-fortified products are the prime examples of it. Addition of iron-containing compounds during the grinding of wheat, otherwise deficient in iron, protects the wheat-dependant populace from diseases caused by deficiency such as iron-deficiency anemias, etc. Iron fortification of wheat has been proven transgenically by expressing phytase gene (*phy*A) from *Aspergillus japonicas* [40]. In situ degradation of phytates in the seed endosperm is considered desirable in order to increase bioavailability of micronutrients [40].

Golden rice and provitamin A-fortified maize are crops that have caught interest of nutritionists globally. Provitamin A deficiency that results in night blindness in masses may be addressed through genetic improvement of crops like maize. In a study where single-cross maize yellow hybrids were evaluated for carotenoid contents [3] since biofortification of maize, endosperm is found to be the most convenient solution addressing its deficiency. Hence, improved contents of provitamin A carotenoids in maize may help Pakistani populace to alleviate the subclinical symptoms of vitamin A deficiency [4].

Perhaps, the most researched aspects of nutraceuticals are their use in medicine, to cure a variety of diseases such as cancer, osteoarthritis, cardiovascular disorders, etc. Over the years, several plants have been shown to contain compounds which, if incorporated into lifestyle early on, reduce the risk of cancer by as much as 33%. For example, blue maize has been found to be an effective nutraceutical in prevention of several types of cancers, such as colon cancer, etc. [41].

This era of rapid urbanization has seen an emerging trend of expressing many medicinal and nutritional traits into other food crops transgenically. Although several people have shown their concerns as to its biosafety, such drawbacks have not been reported to this date. Chloroplast transformation addresses biosafety issues as chloroplasts are not transmitted through pollens in most cultivated plants. Hence, the transgenics are a promising way forward to develop cost-effective nutraceuticals.

4.1.1. Transgenics for therapeutics

A number of pharmaceutical proteins have been synthesized exploiting plant genetic systems with overriding impact on conventional approaches used to manufacture pharmaceuticals. Some advantages of using plant system are low cost of production of pharmaceuticals and their processing. Commercial-scale production in bringing therapeutics to the clinic has been observed in the last 6–7 years. Manufacturing facilities of different capacities have been constructed in addition to the development of plant-made pharmaceuticals to meet current manufacturing standards [42]. Large Scale Biology Corporation (LSBC) in Owensboro, KY, USA, has designed the first manufacturing facility that plant virus transient expression system was developed to meet the current good manufacturing practice [43, 44].

However, synthesizing pharmaceuticals in plants by engineering the chloroplast genome is more advantageous as explained elsewhere in this chapter; therefore, attempts have been made to express different pharmaceuticals proteins. For example, interferons α2 and 5 were expressed from tobacco chloroplasts [5, 6]. In these studies the interferon α2 and 5 genes were synthesized and expressed. It was observed that fully expanded mature leaves contained high levels of interferon hen compared to young and senescence leaves; however, expression levels were very low because of a mutation in the critical region of the promoter during synthesis. Other examples of therapeutic expression are human serum albumin (HSA) that was expressed between 0.02 and 11.1%, depending upon the regulatory sequences used [45], oral and injectable insulin [46], HIV inhibitor cyanovirin [47], TGFb3 [48], and thioredoxins from plastids as modulators of recombinant therapeutic protein production [49]. Recently, different companies and foundations like the Bill and Melinda Gates Foundation or Juvenile Diabetes Research Foundation are undertaking well to advance such developments from labs to the clinics.

4.2. Transgenics for antigenic proteins (vaccines)

Vaccination is an efficient strategy to control viral infections in both human and animal species. Different expression systems, having their own merits and demerits, are being used to produce recombinant vaccines. An ideal system would be that allows producing the desired functional product cost-effectively. Plant-based expression strategies encouraged biotechnologists to use this system to produce vaccines for both humans and animals. Moreover, plant system-derived subunit vaccines are heat stable, bio-encapsulated, and easy to scale up.

Oral vaccine term was introduced and extensively pursued after the successful expression of HBsAg in plants and recovery of the antigen as viruslike particles [50]. Interestingly, the antigen has the same properties as produced in yeast. Later on, the binding subunit of *E. coli* enterotoxin (LTB) and the capsid protein of norovirus genotype, which formed viruslike particles (NV-VLP), was expressed in plants that triggered mucosal immunization response in animals, hence, based on the data on approval clinical trials was obtained [7]. Diverse antigenic proteins were expressed in vegetable and fruit crops, and animal trials were successfully conducted. Plant species used are alfalfa, carrot, lettuce, tomato, potato, maize, soya bean, rice, and banana [51].

Development of an efficient plant-based system to express human antigenic proteins successfully has prompted its application to vaccinate livestock. Different attempts have been made by different research groups to address various diseases of livestock caused by viruses to increase the production in a cost-effective manner. Some of the examples are foot-and-mouth disease virus (FMDV), bovine rotavirus, bovine viral diarrhea virus, bluetongue virus, and bovine papillomavirus. Of these viruses, foot-and-mouth disease virus (FMDV) has been addressed majorly as livestock is an inevitable part of the economy. Livestock productivity is compromised due to frequent occurrence of foot-and-mouth disease (FMD). Vaccination is one of the main strategies to control foot-and-mouth disease. Yet, lack of high-quality and effective vaccine in Pakistan warrants the development of genotype-matched vaccines. One of the approaches to develop such vaccines is reverse genetics that is very costly and laborious. This demands exploring other alternative approaches. Of the alternative approaches, engineering edible plants with the pathogenicity-causing genes is more promising.

An oral vaccine against FMDV was developed by expressing structural protein VP1 in transgenic *Stylosanthes guianensis* [52]. In these experiments, the level of recombinant protein was varied from 0.1 to 0.5% of total soluble protein. These levels were enough to induce a protective systemic antibody response in mice. In another attempt, capsid precursor polypeptide (P1) was expressed in rice, and 0.6–1.3 mg/g of TSP was observed that induced a protective immune response in mice [53]. Further, in mice when vaccinated orally, FMDV-specific mucosal immune responses were detected. However, partial virus clearance after challenge was observed. To address these low-expression problems, chloroplast transformation approach can be used. In a study, VP1 was expressed in tobacco chloroplasts and 2–3% values were recorded [54]. In another study, epitopes (B cell) of structural proteins VP1 and VP4 and of nonstructural proteins 2C and 3D (T cell) were produced in *N. benthamiana* plants using a plant virus expression system [55]. More recently, tandem-linked VP1 proteins of two serotypes, A and O, are expressed in forage crop *Crotalaria juncea* and fed to guinea pigs that produced humoral as well as cell-mediated immune responses [56]. From all these studies and experiments being carried out in the laboratory of the author of this chapter demonstrate that plant-based overexpression of antigenic proteins to control FMDV is an effective way but needs further experimentation to improve efficacy of edible vaccines by engineering epitopic proteins with different adjuvants (Khan MS, unpublished).

5. Conclusions

Nuclear transformation, achieved using microprojectile bombardment or *Agrobacterium* strains, is predominantly carried out to tailor agronomic traits in crops. However, this technology is not successful to transform upland cotton where cells are recalcitrant to regeneration, despite genome mixing through crosses between different genotypes. Biotechnologists rely on this technology though genes escape and pollinate other related crops or weeds, developing weeds or super weeds, respectively. An alternate strategy to develop transgenics is the chloroplast transformation technology since this technology offers natural gene containment, high-level transgene expression with bona fide structures of proteins, and allows all transformation events to be uniform as far as gene integration into the plastome is concerned. High-level gene expression is due to the polyploid nature of chloroplasts in a cell and of plastomes in each chloroplast, biologically active proteins are due to the presence of chaperon proteins, and uniform integration of transgenes into the plastome is due to the homologous recombination. Hence, chloroplast transformation is more suitable for expression of health-related traits in plants rather agronomic in crops. In either case, transgenics should be grown in the field following approved biosafety guidelines and strict stewardship.

Acknowledgements

The corresponding author would like to acknowledge Punjab Agricultural Research Board (PARB) and Higher Education Commission (HEC) for providing funds to MSK for research.

Author details

Muhammad Sarwar Khan[1]* and Kauser Abdulla Malik[2]

*Address all correspondence to: sarwarkhan_40@hotmail.com

1 Center of Agricultural Biochemistry and Biotechnology (CABB), University of Agriculture, Faisalabad, Pakistan

2 Forman Christian College (A chartered University), Lahore, Pakistan

References

[1] Ye X, Al-Babili S, Kloti A, Zhang J, Lucca P, Beyer P, et al. Engineering the provitamin A (beta-carotene) biosynthetic pathway into (carotenoid-free) rice endosperm. Science. 2000;**287**:303-305

[2] Diretto G, Welsch R, Tavazza R, Mourgues F, Pizzichin D, Beyer P, et al. Silencing of beta-carotene hydroxylase increases total carotenoid and beta-carotene levels in potato tubers. BMC Plant Biology. 2007;**7**:11

[3] Maqbool MA, Aslam M, Khan MS, Beshir B, Ahsan M. Evaluation of single cross yellow maize hybrids for agronomic and carotenoid traits. International Journal of Agriculture and Biology. 2017;**19**:1087-1098

[4] Maqbool MA, Aslam M, Beshir A, Khan MS. Breeding for provitamin A biofortification of maize (*Zea mays L.*). Plant Breeding. 2018;**137**:451-469

[5] Nurjis F, Khan MS. Expression of recombinant interferon alpha-2a in tobacco chloroplasts using microprojectile bombardment. The African Journal of Biotechnology. 2011;**10**:17016-17022

[6] Khan MS, Nurjis F. Synthesis and expression of recombinant interferon alpha-5 gene in tobacco chloroplasts, a non-edible plant. Molecular Biology Reports. 2012;**39**:4391-4400

[7] Giorgi C, Franconi R, Rybicki EP. Human papillomavirus vaccines in plants. Expert Review of Vaccines. 2010;**9**:913-924

[8] Khan MS. Plastid genome engineering in plants: Present status and future trends. Molecular Plant Breeding. 2012;**3**:91-102

[9] Cui C, Song F, Tan Y, Zhou X, Zhao W, Ma F, et al. Stable chloroplast transformation of immature scutella and inflorescences in wheat (*Triticum aestivum L.*). Acta Biochimica et Biophysica Sinica. 2011;**43**:284-291

[10] Khan MS, Maliga P. Fluorescent antibiotic resistance marker to track plastid transformation in higher plants. Nature Biotechnology. 1999;**17**:910-915

[11] Lee SM, Kang K, Chung H, Yoo SH, Xu XM, Lee SB, et al. Plastid transformation in the monocotyledonous cereal crop, rice (*Oryza sativa*) and transmission of transgenes to their progeny. Molecular Cell. 2006;**21**:401-410

[12] Khan MS. Tobacco chloroplast transformation using microprojectile bombardment [PhD Diss.]. UK: University of Cambridge; 1997

[13] Hibberd JM, Linley PJ, Khan MS, Gray JC. Transient expression of green fluorescent protein in various plastid types following microprojectile bombardment. The Plant Journal. 1998;**16**:627-632

[14] Khan MS. Utilizing heterologous promoters to express green fluorescent protein from jellyfish in tobacco chloroplasts. Pakistan Journal of Botany. 2001;**33**:43-52

[15] Chen C, Zheng Y, Liu S, Zhong Y, Wu Y, Li J, et al. The complete chloroplast genome of *Cinnamomum camphora* and its comparison with related Lauraceae species. Peer Journal. 2017;**5**:e3820. DOI: 10.7717/peerj.3820

[16] Chumley TW, Palmer JD, Mower JP, Fourcade HM, Calie PJ, Boore JL, et al. The complete chloroplast genome sequence of Pelargonium x hortorum: Organization and evolution of the largest and most highly rearranged chloroplast genome of land plants. Molecular Biology and Evolution. 2006;**23**:2175-2190

[17] Sugiura M. The chloroplast genome. Plant Molecular Biology. 1992;**19**:149-168

[18] Khan MS, Zafar Y, Malik KA. Light that reflects your effort. International Journal of Agriculture and Biology. 2000;**2**:396-399

[19] Cleland WW, Andrews TJ, Gutteridge S, Hartman FC, Lorimer GH. Mechanism of *Rubisco*: The carbamate as general base. Chemical Reviews. 1998;**98**:549-561

[20] Bock R, Khan MS. Taming plastids for a green future. Trends in Biotechnology. 2004;**22**:311-318

[21] Wingler A, Lea PJ, Quick WP, Leegood RC. Photorespiration: Metabolic pathways and their role in stress protection, philos. Philosophical Transactions of the Royal Society B. 2000;**355**:1517-1529

[22] Lin MT, Occhialini A, Andralojc PJ, Parry MA, Hanson MR. A faster *Rubisco* with potential to increase photosynthesis in crops. Nature. 2014;**513**:547-550

[23] Tolbert NE. The C_2 oxidative photosynthetic carbon cycle. Annual Review of Plant Physiology and Plant Molecular Biology. 1997;**48**:1-25

[24] Kebeish R, Niessen M, Thiruveedh K, Bari R, Hirsch H-J, Rosenkranz R, et al. Chloroplastic photorespiratory bypass increases photosynthesis and biomass production in *Arabidopsis thaliana*. Nature Biotechnology. 2007;**25**:593-599

[25] Khan MS. Engineering photorespiration in chloroplasts: A novel strategy for increasing biomass production. Trends in Biotechnology. 2007;**25**:437-440

[26] Yamamoto H, Kurumiya S, Ohashi R, Fujita Y. Oxygen sensitivity of a nitrogenase-like protochlorophyllide reductase from the cyanobacterium *Leptolyngbya boryana*. Plant and Cell Physiology. 2009;**50**:1663-1673

[27] Yamazaki S, Nomata J, Fujita Y. Differential operation of dual protochlorophyllide reductases for chlorophyll biosynthesis in response to environmental oxygen levels in the cyanobacterium *Leptolyngbya boryana*. Plant Physiology. 2006;**142**:911-922

[28] Nazir S, Khan MS. Chloroplast-encoded *chlB* gene from *Pinus thunbergii* promotes root and chlorophyll pigment development in *Nicotiana tabaccum*. Molecular Biology Reports. 2012;**39**:10637-10646

[29] Hibberd JM, Sheehy JE, Langdale JA. Using C_4 photosynthesis to increase the yield of rice–Rationale and feasibility. Current Opinion in Plant Biology. 2008;**11**:228-231

[30] Steinback KE, McIntosh L, Bogorad L, Arntzen CJ. Identification of the triazine receptor protein as a chloroplast gene product. Proceedings of the National Academy of Sciences of the United States of America. 1981;**78**:7463-7467

[31] Fuerst EP, Norman M. Interactions of herbicides with photosynthetic electron transport. Weed Science. 1991;**39**:458-464

[32] Lutz KA, Knapp JE, Maliga P. Expression of bar in the plastid genome confers herbicide resistance. Plant Physiology. 2001;**125**:1585-1590

[33] Kang T-J, Seo J-E, Yang MS. Herbicide resistance of tobacco chloroplasts expressing the bar gene. Molecular Cell. 2003;**16**:60-66

[34] Khan MS, Ali S, Iqbal J. Developmental and photosynthetic regulation of *Bacillus thuringiensis* δ-endotoxin reveals that engineered sugarcane conferring resistance to 'dead heart' contains no toxins in cane juice. Molecular Biology Reports. 2011;**38**:2359-2369

[35] Tabashnik BE, Unnithan GC, Massonb L, Crowder DW, Lia X, Carrierea V. Asymmetrical cross-resistance between bacillus thuringiensis toxins *Cry1Ac* and *Cry2Ab* in pink bollworm. Proceedings of the National Academy of Sciences of the United States of America. 2009;**106**:11889-11894

[36] Brookes G, Barfoot P. Global impact of biotech crops: Environmental effects, 1996-2010. GM Crops and Food: Biotechnology in Agriculture and the Food Chain. 2012;**3**:129-137

[37] Arrieta JG, Enriquez GA, Suarez V, Estevez A, Fernandez ME, Menedez C, et al. Transgenic potato expressing two antifungal proteins. Biotecnologia Aplicada. 1996;**13**:121

[38] Hoshikawa K, Ishihara G, Takahashi H, Nakamura I. Enhanced resistance to gray mold (*Botrytis cinerea*) in transgenic potato plants expressing thionin genes isolated from *Brassicaceae* species. Plant Biotechnology. 2012;**29**:87-93

[39] De Gray G, Rajasekaran K, Smith F, Sanford J, Daniell H. Expression of an antimicrobial peptide via the chloroplast genome to control phytopathogenic bacteria and fungi. Plant Physiology. 2001;**127**:852-862

[40] Abid N, Khatoon A, Maqbool A, Irfan M, Bashir A, Asif I, et al. Transgenic expression of phytase in wheat endosperm increases bioavailability of iron and zinc in grains. Transgenic Research. 2017;**26**:109-112

[41] Guzmán-Gerónimo RI, Alarcón-Zavaleta TM, Oliart-Ros RM, MezaAlvarado JE, Herrera-Meza S, Chávez-Servia JL. Blue maize extract improves blood pressure, lipid profiles, and adipose tissue in high-sucrose diet induced metabolic syndrome in rats. Journal of Medicinal Food. 2017;**20**:110-115

[42] Wirz H, Sauer-Budge AF, Briggs J, Sharpe A, Shu S, Sharon A. Automated production of plant-based vaccines and pharmaceuticals. Journal of Laboratory Automation. 2012;**17**:449-457

[43] Pogue GP, Lindbo JA, Garger SJ, Fitzmaurice WP. Making an ally from an enemy: Plant virology and the new agriculture. Annual Review of Phytopathology. 2002;**40**:45-74

[44] Pogue GP, Vojdani F, Palmer KE, Hiatt E, Hume S, Phelps J, et al. Production of pharmaceutical-grade recombinant aprotinin and a monoclonal antibody product using plant-based transient expression systems. Plant Biotechnology Journal. 2010;**8**:638-654

[45] Millán AF-S, Mingo-Castel A, Miller M, Daniell H. A chloroplast transgenic approach to hyper-express and purify human serum albumin, a protein highly susceptible to proteolytic degradation. Plant Biotechnology Journal. 2003;**1**:71-79

[46] Boyhan D, Daniell H. Low-cost production of proinsulin in tobacco and lettuce chloroplasts for injectable or oral delivery of functional insulin and C-peptide. Plant Biotechnology Journal. 2011;**9**:585-598

[47] Elghabi Z, Karcher D, Zhou F, Ruf S, Bock R. Optimization of the expression of the HIV fusion inhibitor cyanovirin-N from the tobacco plastid genome. Plant Biotechnology Journal. 2011;**9**:599-608

[48] Gisby M, Mellors P, Madesis P, Ellin M, Laverty H, O'Kane S, et al. A synthetic gene increases TGFβ3 accumulation by 75-fold in tobacco chloroplasts enabling rapid purification and folding into a biologically active molecule. Plant Biotechnology Journal. 2011;**9**:618-628

[49] Sanz-Barrio R, Millán AF-S, Corral-Martínez P, Seguí-Simarro JM, Farran I. Tobacco plastidial thioredoxins as modulators of recombinant protein production in transgenic chloroplasts. Plant Biotechnology Journal. 2011;**9**:639-650

[50] Mason HS, Lam DM, Arntzen CJ. Expression of hepatitis B surface antigen in transgenic plants. Proceedings of the National Academy of Sciences of the United States of America. 1992;**89**:11745-11749

[51] Ahmad P, Ashraf M, Younis M, Hu X, Kumar A, Akram NA, et al. Role of transgenic plants in agriculture and biopharming. Biotechnology Advances. 2012;**30**:524-540

[52] Wang DM, Zhu JB, Peng M, Zhou P. Induction of a protective antibody response to FMDV in mice following oral immunization with transgenic *Stylosanthes spp.* as a feed-stuff additive. Transgenic Research. 2008;**17**:1163-1170

[53] Wang Y, Shen Q, Jiang Y, Song Y, Fang L, Xiao S, et al. Immunogenicity of foot-and-mouth disease virus structural polyprotein P1 expressed in transgenic rice. Journal of Virological Methods. 2012;**181**:12-17

[54] Li Y, Sun M, Liu J, Yang Z, Zhang Z, Shen G. High expression of foot-and-mouth disease virus structural protein VP1 in tobacco chloroplasts. Plant Cell Reports. 2006;**25**:329-333

[55] Andrianova EP, Krementsugskaia SR, Lugovskaia NN, Mayorova TK, Borisov VV, Eldarov MA, et al. Foot and mouth disease virus polyepitope protein produced in bacteria and plants induces protective immunity in guinea pigs. Biochemistry (Moscow). 2011;**76**:339-346

[56] Rao JP, Agrawal P, Mohammad R, Rao SK, Reddy GR, Dechamma HJ, et al. Expression of VP1 protein of serotype A and O of foot-and-mouth disease virus in transgenic sunnhemp plants and its immunogenicity for guinea pigs. Acta Virologica. 2012;**56**:91-99

Chapter 2

The Role of Plant Genotype, Culture Medium and *Agrobacterium* on Soybean Plantlets Regeneration during Genetic Transformation

Phetole Mangena

Additional information is available at the end of the chapter

http://dx.doi.org/10.5772/intechopen.78773

Abstract

An efficient and reproducible plant regeneration protocol is essential for genetic manipulation of important crops *in vitro* through *Agrobacterium*-mediated genetic transformation. However, the establishment of such a procedure for recalcitrant legumes like soybean is still a major challenge. Genotype specificity, culture conditions and inefficient recovery of transgenic microshoots are some of the most important factors which requires optimisation before an efficient system of regeneration can be developed. The purpose of this chapter was to provide a review, and report on the varied responses obtained during the assessment of factors that cause recalcitrance during genetic transformation of soybean. *Agrobacterium* infected double cotyledonary-node explants were tested on MS basal culture medium containing combinations of cytokinins-auxins, as well the different concentrations of antibiotics for callus and shoot proliferation. The study showed that, the efficiency of microshoots and callus induction varied widely between cultures and among the genotypes. About 1.0–20.0 and 5.0–20.0% of callus and shoot induction frequency were obtained on cotyledonary explants transformed with *Agrobacterium* compared to more than 60% efficiency obtained in the controls, respectively. This study revealed that, there are some neglected factors playing a crucial role in genetic manipulation, which require optimisation before genetic transformation and *in vitro* regeneration of transgenic plants could be achieved.

Keywords: *Agrobacterium*, callus, double cotyledonary-node explants, genotype, *in vitro* regeneration, shoots, soybean

1. Introduction

Soybean (*Glycine max* L.) is an important leguminous pulse crop grown for the production of oils and proteins. The legumes include cowpea, lentils, peas, peanuts and other pod producing plants that are cultivated commercially or privately for nutritional, pharmaceutical or industrial purposes. These plants have played a crucial role in the traditional diets of many countries including Brazil, China, India and regions in the Middle East and South America [1]. In contrast, many African and European countries do not fully benefit from the subsistent and commercial cultivation of soybean. The less significant role of soybean in these regions may be due to the poor growth conditions. The growth and productivity of this crop has been adversely affected by the biotic and abiotic stress factors [2]. Even though it has the potential to become a major crop in less cultivated regions (Africa and Europe) because of its many uses (as feed, food, etc.), plant modifications to increase yields are highly required [3].

The genetic modification techniques such as the *Agrobacterium*-mediated genetic transformation, electro and chemical cell surface poration or direct protoplast-mediated DNA transfer need to be used to improve the agro-economic traits of this crop in those regions. *Agrobacterium tumefaciens* is a gram-negative soil borne bacterium, which infect dicotyledonous plants, causing a crown gall disease. The crown gall tumour is formed around the wound sites, creating a reservoir for its infestation [4]. The procedure for plant transformation takes advantage of this natural infecting ability to transfer the tumour-inducing plasmid (Ti-plasmid) into hosts. The plasmid DNA is naturally found within the bacterium, and is exploited for transformation with foreign DNA segments of interest obtained from different sources. The genes of interest could be introduced into the host plant's genome during bacterial infection. This phenomenon is known as genetic transformation, whereby the Ti-plasmid expression and integration of the transfer DNA (cloned segment of DNA transferred into hosts) within the host plant genome can also be inherited by the offspring of the host [5].

The first tissue culture based *in vitro* genetic transformation using this approach was reported by Hinchee et al. [6]. Subsequently, numerous reports emerged including those of Chee et al. [7], Yan et al. [8], Shi-Yun [9], Olhoft et al. [10] and Homrich et al. [11] on the use of *A. tumefaciens* to introduce agro-economic traits such as the resistance to pests (*Bt* crops), enhanced protein quality and drought stress tolerance in soybean. This chapter provides a review on the factors affecting *Agrobacterium*-mediated transformation, and gives an account on the outcomes obtained during the valuation of factors that cause recalcitrance during genetic transformation of soybean. The study provides a thorough analysis of the organogenic and phenotypic responses that occur due to the tissue culture conditions and the amenability of genotypes to *Agrobacterium* infection. The application of antimicrobials, plant growth regulators, culture media, bacterial density and the type of explants used influence the transformation efficiency of soybean. Optimised routine strategies in the transformation of soybean are still a prerequisite, since this crop is highly considered recalcitrant.

2. Importance of soybean

Soybean plays a critical role in world agriculture, providing about 40% proteins, 20% oil and 30% carbohydrates contained within the seeds. This crop serves as the cheapest and profitable form of oilseed worldwide for many producers, especially small holder poultry farmers [5]. The industrial processing of this crop to manufacture high protein rich feeds for livestock, pigs and fish farms is growing immensely. The use of soybean in the production of edible oil and biodiesel as a green alternative fuel is also expanding [6]. In human nutrition and health, soybean meals have proved to reduce the cause of several acute and chronic conditions. Messina [1] reported the improvement of body calcium retention lowering urinary calcium excretion after the use of soy-proteins compared to consumption of a mixture of animal proteins. **Table 1** provides information regarding the estimated amount of seed yields used for industrial processing, meal manufacturing and some of the pharmaceutical products derived from soybeans.

Following the drought because of El Nino-related conditions in the sub-Saharan Africa, soybean yield prospects for 2017/2018 have deteriorated, including productions in South America and Southeast Asia. The lowering projections will influence manufacturing and processing of soybean products for many industries and human consumption. Soybeans were also found to contain low fats (approximately 5%), easily modulated trypsin inhibitors and other compounds considered as non-nutritive components. Some of these compounds like phytate were considered to reduce mineral bioavailability of beans but, it has been postulated that phytic acid also lowers the risk of colon and breast cancer [7]. Soybean is considered an excellent source of iron, zinc and folate which serve as essential nutrients and reduce the risk of neural tube defects in humans and promote efficient uptake of vitamin C [8, 9].

Among all the legumes, soybeans are unique because they are a concentrated source of isoflavones that naturally reduce the risk of cancer and heart disease [1]. In addition, soybeans also contain cysteine proteases protein enzymes. These are one of the group of proteolytic enzymes that catalyse the hydrolysis of various polypeptide substrates for the production

	Yield per harvested mt	Total domestic use (mt)	Total soybean export (mt)	World GDP contribution /100%	Soybean food products	Soybean pharmaceutical products	Soybean industrial processing
United States	117.21	53.07	58.79	22.0	Soymilk	Lecithin	Oil
Brazil	114	42.0	67.0	3.0	Tofu	Hydrolysed	Biodisel
Argentina	57.8	44.84	8.50	0.6	Edamame	vegetable	Waxes
China	12.9	95.0	0.15	12.4	Soysouce	protein (HVP)	Solvents
India	11.5	5.45	0.44	3.2	Poultry feeds	Soy proten-	Hydraulic-
Paraguay	10.67	3.7	6.00	0.6	Infant-	concentrate/	fluids
Canada	6.46	-1.00	-1.00	2.4	formulas	Isolates	Adhesives
Other	20.91	-1.00	-1.00	1.7	Natto	Isoflavones	Fibre/Textile

Note: Data was compiled from various sources; including the Soybean Stat Portal, USDA and FAO. Production values were based on the information available in 2016/17 projections. Production level by **Other** refers to estimates of the least soybean producing countries calculated by the Statistic Portal for soybean yield projection 2016 to 2017.mt- on the Table stands for metric tons

Table 1. Soybean producing areas, yield estimates and consumption/processing on industrial scale.

and assembly of proteins that get remobilised or degraded [10]. Proteases are well known for their key role in biochemical processes, implicated for the development and continuation of several diseases. Their role in disease formation, especially during programmed cell death (PCD) involves dismantling of organelles and the different macro molecules required for plant growth and development. They are largely involved in translation and folding of storage proteins, protein remobilisation, signalling controls and at lesser extent for morphogenesis [11].

3. The transformation process

As already indicated, *Agrobacterium*-mediated genetic transformation relies on the natural genetic transfer process causing crown gall disease in plants. This biological method had led to the modification of genomes or addition of genes in various crop plants like maize, cowpea, sunflower, canola and rice [12–16]. The manipulation of *Agrobacterium* by scientists allowed for the transfer of T-DNA without causing tumours in transformed plants. This was achieved by silencing the tumour-inducing genes found on the extrachromosomal plasmid [17]. The transgenes introduced are specifically defined and precisely transformed in the laboratory before being delivered in targeted host plant tissues.

The delivery protocols differ according to species and the purpose of transformation. Thus, the methods for DNA transfer and expression in various plant species are quite varied and their applications in different genotypes always require optimization. This implies that, a tremendous effort still need to be placed on developing more efficient and reproducible transformation procedures. According to Finer and Dhillon [18], *Agrobacterium* is one of the main methods routinely used by many laboratories for plant transformation. This method is considered rapid, most efficient and cheaper for the transformation of many crop plants compared to other techniques. Other methods used for genetic transformation, their advantages and setbacks are discussed below.

3.1. Other methods of genetic manipulation

One of the most interesting techniques for DNA transfer is Agroinfiltration. In agroinfiltration, *Agrobacterium* is infiltrated or injected into plant cells (leaves) of a suitable host. This method induces transient expression of genes in a plant by forcing *Agrobacterium* suspension into the internal leaf tissues using a syringe [19]. Zhao et al. [20] reported transformation of *Nicotiana benthamiana* using this method with *Agrobacterium* strain harbouring pCAMBIA1301. The β-glucuronidase (GUS) expression and GUS activity showed increased transgene expression more than 6-fold for agroinfiltration suspension containing 20 μM 5-azacytidine, 0.56 mM ascorbic acid and 0.03% Tween-20. The floral dip method of *Agrobacterium*-mediated transformation also have been developed. The flowers of plants to be transformed are immersed in a suspension of *Agrobacterium* containing wetting agent, for example; Tween-20 or Silwet to allow bacterial access to pores or cracks on the flower. This method was reported by Finer and Dhillon [18] to be designed specifically for *Arabidopsis*, and there is no other plant that, currently respond positively like *Arabidopsis*. In contrast, Verma et al. [21] reported more than 1% transformation efficiency in *Brassica napus* cv. Elect and *Brassica carinata* cv. Pusa Gaurav using this method. However, various attempts in many plant species to develop floral dip transformation protocols have been met with very limited transformation efficiencies [21]. Another method is particle bombardment invented by John Sanford [22]. This microprojectile or biolistic bombardment employs particle acceleration coated DNA into the target plant tissues. Once in the cells, the DNA becomes permanently integrated into the chromosomes of the host plant genome [20]. Although, there are numerous techniques used for transformation, all methods face the same challenges of inefficiency, lack of a routinely used protocol and the genotype specificity problem.

3.2. Challenges faced during genetic transformation

There are several challenges faced during the process of delivering segments of oncogenic DNA to susceptible plant cells. The limitations are mostly associated with *in vitro* culture conditions than the genetic transfer and expression. Plant regeneration *in vitro* can be efficiently and rapidly achieved for plantlets micropropagation. Soybean has been successfully regenerated through adventitious/axillary/meristem shoot organogenesis and direct or indirect somatic embryogenesis using different types of mature and immature explants. But, coupling *in vitro* plant tissue culture with transformation to improve production of transgenic plants presents its own challenges. To produce transformants, especially in soybeans, *in vitro* culturing strategies that are highly efficient are required. Soybean is still considered a recalcitrant crop, and the nature of culture media and susceptibility of selected explants to *Agrobacterium* influences transgenic plant regeneration efficiency.

Constraining factors such as; genotype specificity, antibiotics toxicity, selection pressure, explant type and age, *Agrobacterium* overgrowth and contaminations are still being neglected. Zia [23] indicated that, these abovementioned factors play a key developmental role in *in vitro* manipulation of plants. Failure of many tissue culture based *in vitro* transformations is mainly due to these factors. In addition, other forms of transformation like electroporation, particle bombardment and protoplast-mediated transformation pose more challenges than *Agrobacterium*-mediated genetic transformation under *in vitro* culture conditions. These techniques are expensive to carry-out, are labour intensive with prolonged steps of transformation, cause unstable transgene expression particularly due to gene silencing [24], produce multiple transgene copy number [12] and cause gene rearrangement within inserts and instability over the generation of transgenic plants [25].

4. Role of genetic transformation in soybean improvement

Plant transformation has become the most important and reliable technology for the improvement of many crop cultivars, as well as for studying gene functions in plants. In soybean, the technique has already been used to produce genetically modified plants. The genetically modified soybeans range from metabolically engineered plants such as those exhibiting increased oleic acid as well as the herbicide-tolerant (HT) cultivars [26, 27]. Soybean transformation led to production of elite cultivars, increased gene pool, plants with improved secondary metabolites and production of disease free plants, especially regenerated under aseptic culture conditions [2, 28]. As the attempts in soybean transformation progresses, procedures must focus on transgenic plant production exhibiting tolerance to abiotic stress factors. This is so, because soybean growth and productivity is severely hampered by abiotic stress, particularly drought. Drought refers to the absence of rainfall or irrigation for a period sufficient to deplete soil moisture to a level not sustaining plant growth [29]. The decrease in water content completely arrest cell functioning, including the support to plant cell and tissue metabolism, meiotic/mitotic division and differentiation. Some of the reports that have assessed the severity of drought on soybean growth include those of Heatherly [30], Desclaux et al. [31] and Brown et al. [32]. Studies continue to show that the GM soybean varieties have important applications, including the use in biodiesel production. Increased yield emanating from genetic improvement is required for the production of more soybean oil used for manufacturing of biodiesel. Besides the utilisation of soybean oil as a major feedstock for biodiesel production [33], the hull can be used to manufacture ethanol from the significant amount of carbohydrates it contains [34]. All these reports clearly indicate the importance of transformation in increasing yield quantity of high quality. According to Zia [23] and Yu et al. [35] transgenic soybean cultivars account for more than 85% of cultivars cultivated for commercial production worldwide, and the cultivars used still require traits improvements.

5. Tissue culture-based transformation

The success of *Agrobacterium*-mediated genetic transformation is largely due to the correct optimisation of culture conditions, each manipulated by media modification and environmental control. Four (4) main factors were recognised in this study for the improvement of genetic transformation under *in vitro* plant tissue culture. The specific factors are:

- Culture medium conditions
- Plant genotype
- Type of explant
- *Agrobacterium* strain and density

The establishment of aseptic *in vitro* culture conditions usually includes the culture medium with basal inorganic nutrient elements (both micro- and macro- elements), organic energy source (primarily sucrose) and the vitamins. Culture media are furthermore, semi-solidified with agar or other commercially available gelling agents, like the gelrite [36]. Precisely defined *in vitro* culture media and other conditions are required for exploitation in the initiation and induction of different cultures from genetically engineered tissues. In this study, defined media compositions were designed to assess the effects of media and *Agrobacterium* suspension on the regeneration of transformed soybean plantlets (**Table 2**). This was done for the seed cultures used to establish seedlings, to develop the double cotyledonary-node explants, infection of explants with *Agrobacterium*, co-culturing medium and regeneration of multiple adventitious shoots. Procedures used for the preparation of *Agrobacterium tumefaciens* inoculum and co-cultivation of explants was conducted as described by Paz et al. [37] with modifications.

Culture modifications included, reduced infection period (15 min immersion of explants in the infection medium), increased amounts of antibiotics used for washing of infected double coty-node explants following co-cultivation with *Agrobacterium* (200 mgL^{-1} cefotaxime and

Macro- elements	Amount (mg/l)	Micro- elements	Amount (mg/l)	Organic additives	Amount (mg/l)
NH_4NO_3	1650	H_3BO_3	6.2	Glycine	2
KNO_3	1900	$MnSO_4$	22.3	Myoinositol	100
$CaCl_2.7H_2O$	440	$ZnSO_4.2H_2O$	0.25	Nicotinic acid	0.5
$MgSO_4.7H_2O$	370	KI	0.83	Thiamine HCl	0.5
FeEDTA	35	$Na_2MoO_4.2H_2O$	0.25	Pyridoxine	0.5
KH_2PO_4	170	$CuSO_4.5H_2O$	0.25	Sucrose	30000
		$CoSO_4.7H_2O$	0.03	Gelrite (Gellan gum)	2500

Culture medium, plant growth regulators (PGRs) and other culture support systems

Germination medium	MS basal culture medium and 4.0 mgL^{-1} 6-benzylaminopurine (6-BA), pH 5.8
Infection medium	Gamborg's B5 basal medium, methyl ester sulfonate (MES), gibberellic acid (GA_3), 6-BA and acetosyringone at pH 5.4 (Paz et al., 2006).
Co-cultivation medium	B5 basal medium, MES, agar, GA_3, 6-BA, cysteine, dithiothreitol (DTT), and acetosyringone, at pH 5.4 (Paz et al., 2006).
Shoot induction medium	MS basal medium, 2.0 mgL-1 6-BA, 8.0 mgL^{-1} glufosinate, 50 mgL^{-1} vancomycin and 100 mgL^{-1} cefotaxime at pH 5.8.
Shoot elongation	PGRs free MS basal medium, 8.0 mgL^{-1} glufosinate, 50 mgL^{-1} vancomycin and 100 mgL^{-1} cefotaxime at pH 5.8.
Rooting medium	MS basal medium, 8.0 mgL^{-1} glufosinate, 2.70 mgL^{-1} indole-3-butyric acid (IBA) and 2.30 mgL^{-1} naphthalene acetic acid (NAA), 50 mgL^{-1} vancomycin and 100 mgL^{-1} cefotaxime at pH 5.8.

Note: Gamborg's B5 and MS basal media were prepared according to Pierik [37]

Table 2. Modified Gamborg's B5 and MS basal culture media used for *in vitro Agrobacterium*-mediated genetic transformation of soybean using double cotyledonary-node explants derived from 10-day old seedlings.

200 mgL^{-1} vancomycin), reduced co-cultivation period of 3-days and high concentrations of DTT and L-cysteine in the co-cultivation medium. These factors were modified to improve the transformation efficiency, particularly using aseptic culture conditions to stimulate proliferative capacity of explants and influence the explant viability. Given the current figure of less than 10% transformation efficiency so far achieved, there is no doubt that established protocols still need to be improved.

5.1. Double cotyledonary-nodes preparation and co-cultivation

The use of double cotyledonary-node explants derived from seedlings germinated on MS medium for *in vitro* regeneration and transformation of soybeans have been previously reported [38]. In this study, the coty-node explants were also prepared from 10-day old soybean seedlings developed from MS basal culture medium supplemented with 4.0 mgL^{-1} 6-BA as indicated on **Table 2**. Seedlings of soybean cultivar Dundee, LS 677, LS 678, TGx 1740-2F, TGx 1835-10E and Peking were transversely cut on the hypocotyl segments, 5–8 mm beneath cotyledons and their epicotyls excised from the base, at cotyledonary junctions to produce double cotyledonary-node explants. The explants comprised of the embryonic axis, section of the hypocotyl and two cotyledons. All coty-nodes were placed with their abaxial side down on the culture media and used for establishment of callus and shoots cultures. A total of 60 double cotyledonary-node explants were prepared for each set of replicates, and the procedure was repeated four times for all transformation cultures.

5.2. Callus induction

A full-strength MS culture media containing macronutrients, micronutrients and vitamins, 3% sucrose, as well as 0.25% gelrite were used in this study. The different concentrations and combinations of PGRs were added into the media from prepared stock solutions made by dissolving analytical reagent grade hormones with few drops of 1 N sodium hydroxide and making-up the final volume with distilled water. The medium used to test for the efficiency of callus initiation on double coty-nodes infected with *A. tumefaciens* containing the *oc-1* gene on pTF101.1 vector contained 0.70 mgL^{-1} kinetin (KI), 2.70 mgL^{-1} indole-3-butyric acid (IBA) and 3.20 mgL^{-1} α-naphthalene acetic acid (NAA). Another medium was supplemented with 0.50 mgL^{-1} KI, 1.20 mgL^{-1} IBA and 1.20 mgL^{-1} NAA. The media and hormonal compositions selected and reported in this chapter induced the best callus initiation and development, and were selected from findings made during preliminary studies.

A. tumefaciens strain EHA 101 constituting vector construct pTF101.1 used for transformation of cotyledonary explants was re-initiated, centrifuged and pelleted (OD_{650} = 0.6–0.8) as described by Paz et al. [37]. The bacterium was resuspended in liquid infection medium prepared as indicated on **Table 2**. Prepared soybean explants were then added into the infection medium and incubated at room temperature for 15-min with gentle shaking on an orbital shaker (Orbishake-Labotec). After infection, the explants were briefly rinsed and then placed on co-cultivation medium containing B5 chemicals (major salts, minor salts, vitamins and iron source), 30 gL^{-1} sucrose, 3.9 gL^{-1} MES, 4.25 gL^{-1} agar, at pH 5.4. Filter sterilised 0.25 mgL^{-1} GA_3, 400 mgL^{-1} cysteine, 200 mgL^{-1} dithiothreitol (DTT) and 50 mgL^{-1} acetosyringone were added into the medium after autoclaving. Co-cultivation of explants was carried-out by incubation in a culture room for 3-days at 24 ± 2°C under 50–60 μmolm^{-2} s^{-2} light intensity with 16-h photoperiod. Later, these *Agrobacterium* infected explants were cultured on callus induction medium supplemented with different concentrations of growth regulators as indicated above.

5.2.1. *Effect of culture media, explant infection and genotypes on callus induction*

The results obtained in this study indicated that aseptically developed seedlings were necessary for callus initiation. Seed germination as measured by protrusion of the root radicle was achievable from the 3rd day of incubation. Seed cultures were maintained in the culture room for 10-days to achieve more than 75% seed germination. Variations in the percentage germination were also observed, with cultivar LS 678 recording 98% germination followed by TGx 1835-10E, LS 677, Dundee, TGx 1740-2F and Peking with 95, 84, 80, 82 and 78% germination respectively. Successful seed germination has proved essential for many *in vitro* culture developments. This initial step has been reported by El-Kaaby et al. [39] and Bahry et al. [40] as a good indicator of seed viability and therefore, a determinant of the success to be achieved in plant tissue culture. According to the prescriptions by the International Seed Testing Association (ISTA), seeds should prove to be viable by ultimately achieving more than 60% overall germination percentage. This study, including other previous studies indicated that, reduced seed viability negatively affects seedling vigour required for successful initiation of shoots and callus cultures.

Given the good and viable explants used in this study, the results obtained during callus cultures showed that, callus induction was achievable using the chosen MS medium and the different kinds of plant growth regulators (KI, IBA and NAA) used. However, the MS medium, together with the hormonal combinations resulted in significant amounts of callus cells in the controls than on explants infected with *Agrobacterium*. Variations in the amount/size of the callus and calli phenotypes were also observed. Generally, very little callus cells were observed from cotyledonary nodes transformed with *Agrobacterium*. But, more compact, embryogenic and friable callus cells were observed from culture medium supplemented with different combinations of KI, IBA and NAA without explant co-cultivation with the bacterium. The infection of explants influenced explant survival and responsiveness in addition to the callus induction capacity as illustrated in **Table 3**. The results indicated that, MS media containing antibiotics also delayed callus initiation. This was confirmed when un-transformed explants were subcultured on a media containing antibiotics. Callus initiation was arrested for more than 3 weeks of culture. But later, swelling and traces of slightly white-yellow friable callus was observed on the explants. The few small masses of callus rapidly turned brownish to ultimately black in colour (**Figure 1**). Zhang et al. [41] made similar observations when investigating the effect of kanamycin in tissue culture and induction of somatic embryos in cotton. This direct organogenesis of callus reported reduction of callus initiation and growth on medium supplemented with 10 mgL^{-1} of kanamycin. The study furthermore, reported complete inhibition of callus formation in medium supplemented with 60 mgL^{-1} concentration of kanamycin.

Paz et al. [37] reported prophylactic and proliferative effects in soybean culture using 100 mgL^{-1} cefotaxime and 50 mgL^{-1} vancomycin. Even though, Grzebelus and Skop [42] shared similar sentiments to Paz et al. [37] when investigating the effect of β-lactams antimicrobials on *in vitro* carrot protoplast culture, the formation of callus on medium amended with these antibiotics was negatively affected. They evaluated three types of β-lactams (cefotaxime, carbenicillin and timentin) at five different concentrations (100, 200, 300 or 500 mgL^{-1}), which were higher than what was used in this study. The low levels of callus and poor explant competency observed in this study, on infected and un-infected explants, can be largely attributed to the presence of antibiotics in the medium used (**Figure 2**). However, a dual negative effect was exerted on the cultures by both *Agrobacterium* infection and media composition, particularly on the proliferation from cotyledonary-node explants. The level of explant competency on these cultures appeared profoundly negatively affected compared to nearly 100% callus induction efficiencies obtained in all genotypes for both proembryonic masses and large size formations in the controls (**Table 3**). According to **Figure 2**, the media, PGRs concentration selected and explants were successful in inducing callus as supported by Barwale et al. [43] and Franklin and Dixon [44].

The media compositions directed the development of plant cells in the cultures by essentially influencing the plasticity and totipotency of the plant tissues used as explants. This observation is in line with many studies, especially demonstrating the synergic effects of auxin (IBA, NAA) and cytokinin (KI) combination used in this study. All cultivars produced some callus on MS medium containing 0.7 mgL^{-1} KI, 2.7 mgL^{-1} IBA and 3.2 mgL^{-1} NAA as indicated in **Table 3**, in relation to **Table 2**. The results observed on MS-A and MS-B culture medium formulations could also be linked to the soybean cultivars used. Plant tissue swelling and initiation of calli was observed within a week of culture in more than 50% replicates of all

Infected explants- MS medium A				Un-infected control- MS medium A		
	Callus induction frequency (%)	Callus type	Callus colour	Callus induction frequency (%)	Callus type	Callus colour
Dundee	6.67*	compact	brown	70.5*	Friable/compact	White-yellow
LS 677	13.33*	compact	brown	88.8*	Friable/compact	White-yellow
LS 678	8.33*	compact	brown	90.0*	Friable/compact	White-yellow
TGx 1740-2F	1.0^{ns}	compact	---	74.5*	Friable/compact	White-brownish
TGx 1835-10E	1.0^{ns}	compact	---	65.5*	Mostly compact	White-brownish
Peking	20.0*	slightly friable	white/brown	85.5*	Mostly friable	White-yellowish
Infected explants- MS medium B				**Un-infected control- MS medium B**		
Dundee	3.33^{ns}	compact	brown	65.0*	Compact	White-brownish
LS 677	---	---	---	74.0*	Friable/compact	White-yellow
LS 678	3.33^{ns}	compact	brown	66.5*	Friable/compact	White-yellow
TGx 1740-2F	---	---	---	55.0*	Friable/compact	White-brownish
TGx 1835-10E	---	---	---	45.0*	Friable/compact	White-brownish
Peking	10.0*	compact	brown	70.5*	Friable/compact	White-brownish

Note: Evaluation was carried out after 4 weeks of culture. Percentage on callus induction frequency was calculated as (total number of explants inducing callus without shoots or roots/ total cultured explants) x 100%. All values within the column are the mean values calculated from 60 replicates per cultivar. Values with asterisks are significantly different and values with ns are not significant at 5% confidence level using t-test. The experiments were repeated four times. MS medium A- is medium supplemented with 0.70 mgL-1 KI, 2.70 mgL-1 IBA and 3.20 mgL-1 NAA. MS medium B- is medium supplemented with 0.50 mgL-1 KI, 1.20 mgL-1 IBA and 1.20 mgL-1 NAA.

Table 3. The response of un-infected coty-node explants and *Agrobacterium tumefaciens* infected double cotyledonary-node explants on callus induction in soybean.

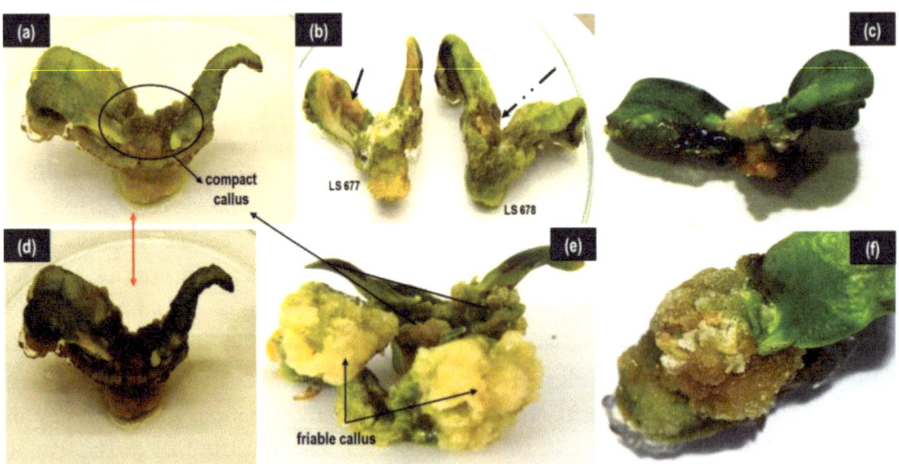

Figure 1. Double cotyledonary-nodes showing callus induction on infected and un-infected explants. (a, d) Failure of callus formation on a coty-node infected with *A. tumefaciens*. (b) White-yellow and brownish callus induced on MS medium containing antibiotics using un-infected explants. (c) Callus and shoot formed on un-infected explant subcultured on MS medium containing KI (0.70 mgL^{-1}), IBA (2.70 mgL^{-1}) and NAA (3.20 mgL^{-1}). (e, f) Callus formation on un-infected explants subcultured on MS medium containing KI (0.50 mgL^{-1}), IBA (1.20 mgL^{-1}) and NAA (1.20 mgL^{-1}).

genotypes. The induced callus culture grew into significantly large amount of callus, particularly in the controls, while maintaining their morphological potential. Callus initiation and cell multiplication for example; in soybean cultivar LS 678 and Peking responded rapidly

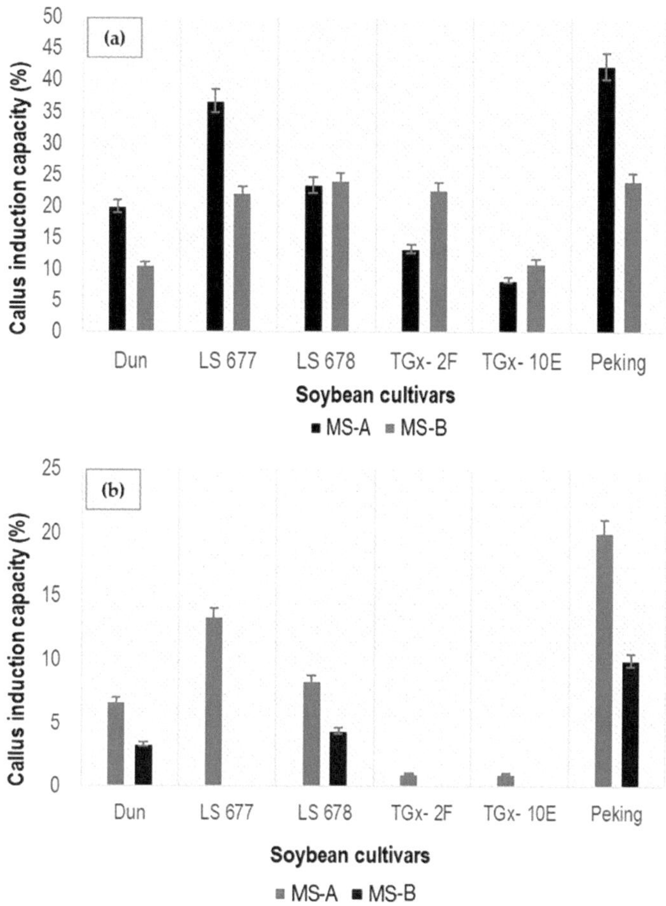

Figure 2. Callus induction capacity on double cotyledonary-node explants on MS medium A (KI- 0.70 mgL^{-1}, IBA-2.70 mgL^{-1} and NAA-3.20 mgL^{-1}) and MS medium B (KI-0.50 mgL^{-1}, IBA-1.20 mgL^{-1} and NAA-1.20 mgL^{-1}). (a) callus induction on un-infected explants subcultured on MS-A (black bar) and MS-B (grey bar) containing antibiotics. (b) callus induction on infected explants subcultured on MS-A (grey bar) and MS-B (black bar) containing antibiotics.

to the culture conditions than any other genotypes. Furthermore, MS-A induced the largest amount of callus in cultivar LS 677, LS 678, Dundee, TGx 1740-2F, TGx 1835-10E and Peking consecutively than MS-B culture medium.

TGx 1835-10E produced the largest amount of chlorophyll callus and exhibited considerably high frequency of shoot and root organogenesis than TGx 1740-2F. Cultivar Peking on the other hand, produced clumps of callus cells on the cotyledon margins, junction and exhibited some browning of the cells at the bases of the hypocotyls as indicated in **Figure 3**.

The cotyledonary-node explants exhibited progressive chlorosis and necrosis after 3 weeks of culture for both MS medium A and B. Generally, inhibitory effects on explant swelling for formation of plant callus tissues was more pronounced on infected tissues and explants sub-cultured on media containing antibiotics. These results clearly demonstrated the effects that all factors examined have on callus initiation and development, as well as morphogenesis, including potential organogenesis in *in vitro* culture of soybean.

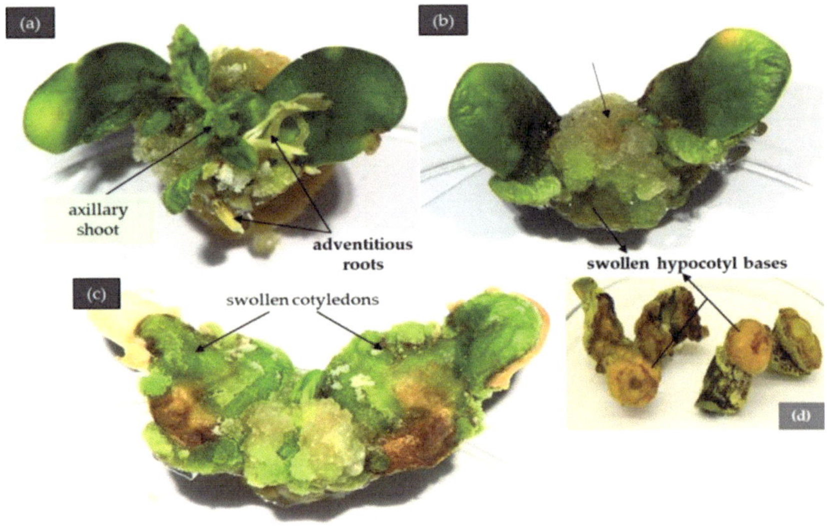

Figure 3. Examples of root and shoot organogenesis and swollen nodes, on explants subcultured for callus induction using MS-B. (a) Rooting and shoot initiation occurring during callus culture. (b) Induced friable callus. (c) Swollen cotyledons. (d) Swelling on hypocotyl segments.

5.3. Shoot multiplication

The development of an efficient protocol for *Agrobacterium*-mediated genetic transformation in soybean is important for improving the genetic pool of this crop. Soybean is considered recalcitrant to genetic manipulation, and its *in vitro* based protocols are faced with many challenges. The following results summarises the influence that factors such as; the genotype, explant type, culture media and *Agrobacterium* infection have on the optimisation of efficient shoot induction during *in vitro* transformation procedures.

5.3.1. Response of explants to culture medium and Agrobacterium infection

Shoot induction was achievable on the MS media compositions used in this study. More than 60% of the coty-node explants proliferated adventitious shoots within 2-weeks of culture on MS medium supplemented with 2.0 mgL^{-1} 6-BA. According to the results, the highest number of shoots was obtained on all MS media containing 2.0 mgL^{-1} of 6-BA and un-infected explants used as a control. MS medium further supplemented with cefotaxime and vancomycin (**Table 2**) also successfully induced a significant number of multiple shoots. Generally, sufficient shoot induction was achievable using cotyledonary nodes without co-cultivation with *Agrobacterium* on MS medium supplemented either with antibiotics or without antibiotics (**Table 4**). Shoot formation on transformed explants was highly reduced (**Table 4**), probably because of the combined inhibitory effects of bacterial infection and antibiotics as described during callus induction.

A small number of shoots on un-infected explants was induced on medium containing antibiotics compared to the MS medium without antibiotics. Most of these explants initiated highly reduced shoots and multiple buds without promotion to further growth. In contrast, intact and elongated multiple shoots were observed, ranging between 3 and 5 shoots on average for MS

Culture Media without Antibiotics				Culture Media with Antibiotics			
Cultivar	Mean shoot ± Std. Error	Std. Deviation	Variance	Cultivar	Mean shoot ± Std. Error	Std. Deviation	Variance
	Uninfected coty-node explants				Uninfected coty-node explants		
Dundee	3.850 ± 0.274	1.226	1.503*	Dundee	1.350 ± 0.221	0.988	0.976*
LS 677	4.450 ± 0.344	1.538	2.366	LS 677	1.750 ± 0.216	0.967	0.934
LS 678	4.650 ± 0.372	1.663	2.766*	LS 678	1.950 ± 0.185	0.826	0.682
TGx 1740-2F	3.400 ± 0.336	1.501	2.253*	TGx 1740-2F	1.150 ± 0.150	0.671	0.450*
TGx 1835-10E	4.450 ± 0.394	1.762	3.103*	TGx 1835-10E	0.750 ± 0.190	0.851	0.724*
Peking	5.000 ± 0.384	1.717	2.947	Peking	1.350 ± 0.109	0.489	0.239*
					Explants infected with *Agrobacterium*		
				Dundee	1.250 ± 0.270	1.209	1.461*
				LS 677	1.400 ± 0.328	1.465	2.147
				LS 678	1.400 ± 0.328	1.465	2.147*
				TGx 1740-2F	0.750 ± 0.216	0.967	0.934*
				TGx 1835-10E	0.800 ± 0.156	0.696	0.484*
				Peking	1.650 ± 0.335	1.496	2.239*

Note: Mean values accompanied with an asterisk* within columns are significantly different at p value = 0.05 confidence level. Values within columns without asterisks are not statistically significant at the given p value according to the t-test.

Table 4. Comparison of the effect of MS basal culture media with or without antibiotics and *Agrobacterium* infection of double cotyledonary-node explants on average number of shoots induced per explant after 30 days of culture.

medium without antibiotics (**Table 4**). The suppression of shoot initiation and growth clearly appears to be instigated by the presence of antibiotics in the medium than the genotype factor. These observations confirmed the findings made in the previous section on callus induction. The initiation and proliferation of callus evidently relied upon the presence of antibiotics in the culture medium. Similar results were obtained by Yu et al. [45], when assessing the effects of carbenicillin and cefotaxime on callus and somatic embryogenesis from adventitious roots of papaya, as previously indicated. The report indicated extreme inhibitory effect of these antibiotics on callus growth, and reported abnormalities on somatic embryos generated on culture medium supplemented with 250–500 mgL^{-1} carbenicillin and cefotaxime.

The cotyledonary-nodes subcultured on MS basal medium with only 2.0 mgL^{-1} 6-BA, without antibiotics induced the highest significant number of shoots within 2 weeks of culture (**Table 4**). Vigorous shoot growth, as indicated in **Figure 4a** and **b**, was obtained on this medium and the initiated microshoots reached elongation, rooting and acclimatisation stages successfully. Generally, variations in culture were observed among the basal media and infected cultures in the percentage of explants forming shoots and mean number of shoots induced per explant. Shoot induction dynamics similar to this observation were reported by El-Siddig et al. [46] and Yan et al. [47]. The transformation trials in these studies revealed great differences in the regeneration frequency, which mostly depended on the explant type and the culture conditions, particularly the culture media compositions. In this study, the results showed that morphogenetic processes are strongly influenced by the culture media, predominantly the presence of antibiotics in the medium.

The requirement of suitable explants for soybean regeneration *in vitro* is one of the main goals leading to efficacious genetic transformation. The use of double cotyledonary-nodes still shows superiority, with greater potential on the development of a simple and effective genetic manipulation protocol. These explants withstood the culture conditions used and provided a feasible mean of culture establishment. The double coty-node explants in addition, offer prolonged

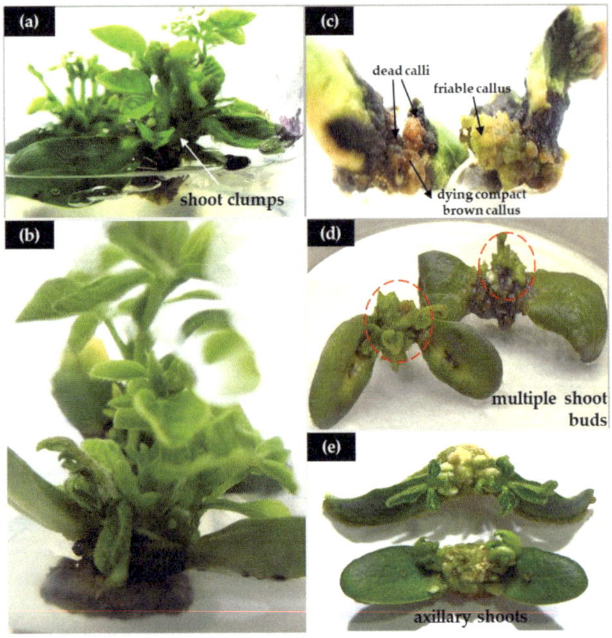

Figure 4. Shoot induction from double-cotyledonary node explants on MS culture medium supplemented with 2.0 mgL^{-1} 6-BA. (a, b) Shoot multiplication on un-infected coty-node explants cultured on MS medium used as control without antibiotics. (c) Callus formation and senescence from cotyledonary-nodes cultured on MS medium containing cefotaxime and vancomycin antibiotics. (d) Shoot buds initiated on explants infected with *Agrobacterium*. (e) Shoots initiated with on explants cultured on medium containing antibiotics without *Agrobacterium* infection.

support to shoots and buds initiated on the cotyledonary junction and exhibit minimal deficiency symptoms on their cotyledons. Even though, these explants show little sensitivity to culture conditions compared to the hypocotyl segments or immature cotyledons as indicated by Zhang et al. [41], their response was much better, especially subsequent *Agrobacterium* infection. The shoots and buds appeared to be well and effectively supported by these explants. Double cotyledonary-node explants produced better responses than the use of single coty-node explants. These single coty-nodes are prepared by longitudinally splitting the double coty-nodes at the cotyledonary junction into two single nodes [38]. Even if high proliferation of shoots can be achieved on other types of explants by directly stimulating pre-existing axillary meristems and induce rapid cell division because of severe wounding, tissue senescence due to bacterium overgrowth and callus formation instead of shoots still make double coty-nodes preferable than single coty-nodes.

6. *In vitro* regeneration of transgenic shoots

Transgenic shoot proliferation and multiplication are not easily achieved from the meristematic regions of the *Agrobacterium* infected double cotyledonary-node explants. This is the case, even if shoot development may be stimulated by the removal of the epicotyls during explant preparation and incisions on pre-determined axillary meristematic cells found on the cotyledonary junctions. In this study, tissue browning caused by oxidation and accumulation of phenolic compounds affected shoot initiation (**Figures 1d** and **4c** and **d**). More than 50%

http://dx.doi.org/10.5772/intechopen.78773

Source of Variation	Explants forming shoot buds (%)	Shoot induction frequency (%)	Regeneration frequency (%)
Culture medium with antibiotics			
Dundee	55.00^c	15.00^d	0.91^*
LS 677	60.00^b	30.05^c	2.70^*
LS 678	55.00^c	35.20^b	.
TGx 1740-2F	45.00^d	5.05^e	.
TGx 1835-10E	65.00^a	.	.
Peking	65.00^a	40.05^a	5.23^*
***Agrobacterium* infected explants**			
Dundee	75.5^e	10.0^c	.
LS 677	80.0^d	15.0^b	0.31^*
LS 678	90.5^b	20.0^a	.
TGx 1740-2F	85.0^c	0.0^e	.
TGx 1835-10E	55.5^f	5.00^d	.
Peking	100.0^a	0.00^e	.
Culture without antibiotics/infected explants			
Dundee	100.0^a	85.0^c	77.70^*
LS 677	100.0^a	95.6^b	80.03^*
LS 678	100.0^a	80.5^d	78.60
TGx 1740-2F	95.0^b	75.0^e	57.32^*
TGx 1835-10E	100.0^a	85.0^c	67.91^*
Peking	100.0^a	100.0^a	83.70^*

NOTE: Values within columns designated by same alphabets are not statistically different at 1% confidence level. Values accompanied by asterisks are significantly different at p-value less than 0.05%. **Explants forming buds (%)** was calculated from the mean number of shoots inducing shoot buds, **Shoot induction frequency (%)** was determined from the mean number of explants inducing more than three or more shoots per explant, and % **regeneration frequency** is calculated from the mean number of shoots per cultivar reaching rooting and acclimatisation stages.

Table 5. The response of soybeans to modified MS culture media and infection with *Agrobacterium tumefaciens* constituting a pTF101.1 vector.

of explants exhibiting shoot growth inhibition due to oxidative browning induced compact callus. This had negative effects on the rate of shoot and thus, the regeneration of transformed microshoots was dramatically decreased in all cultures tested for *Agrobacterium*-mediated genetic transformation. All soybean genotypes used in this study had been affected by oxidative browning, despite modifying the medium according prescriptions made in the literature. Several approaches have been reported, such as; the addition of dithiothreitol, polyvinylpyrrolidone (PVP), activated charcoal and other antioxidant mixtures like ascorbic acid. Jones and Saxena [48] report a novel approach of introducing PAL inhibitor, inhibiting the activity of phenyl-alanine ammonia lysate (PAL) enzyme. This enzyme catalyses the formation of phenolic compounds through phenylpropanoid metabolic pathway. However, shoot induction frequency of all cultivars ranged between 0.0 and 20% as indicated in **Table 5**. Only 0.31% regeneration frequency was obtained in LS 677 (**Table 5**). The detrimental effect of oxidative stress on the number of shoots induced per explants, induced shoots growth and transformation efficiency was also reported by Li et al. [49]. This problem has been correspondingly reported to have affected the efficiency of many cultures in plant tissue organogenesis and embryogenesis. For example; Hartmann et al. [50] reported failure to achieve *in vitro* plantlets regeneration during mass propagation of non-transgenic plants.

7. The role of genotype in soybean transformation

Several studies including those of Zhang et al. [51], Yan et al. [47], Paz et al. [52] and Li et al. [49] have showed that genetic transformation in soybean is highly genotype specific. According to the results in **Tables 4** and **5**, cultivar TGx 1740-2F and TGx 1835-10E were highly recalcitrant. These cultivars showed consistent difficulties for callus and shoot proliferation under used culture conditions. Consecutively, the highest number of shoots were induced in soybean cv. Peking, LS 677 and LS 678. This was followed by cultivar Dundee and lastly, the two TGx varieties. These soybeans gave the same morphogenic trend when cultured for *in vitro* regeneration in the controls. The reports cited above support this study by concurring with the findings made in this study. The generation of reactive oxygen species upon *Agro*-infection of explants leading to oxidative browning and subsequent tissue browning was also more prevalent in Dundee, TGx 1740-2F and TGx 1835-10E genotypes. The intensity of explant tissue browning and necrosis is a key indicator of explant proliferative or totipotency potential. However, the continued testing of different types and concentrations of antioxidants such as DTT may minimise cell necrosis and improve the transformation frequencies in soybean.

The ability of genotypes to resist the influence of modified culture conditions aimed at regenerating new plants have been widely reported. Thirty-eight cultivars of *Gossypium* showed high, moderated, low and non-somatic embryogenic response under different regime of plant growth regulators. The level of responses did not change and genotypic variation for embryogenesis was found to exist as indicated by Trolinder and Xhixian [53]. Relatively low breeding progress, high self-incompatibility and inbreeding depression may be some of the factors encouraging genotype specificity and recalcitrance in many crops. Evidence of these effects were reported by Gawali et al. [54], Targonska et al. [55], Nguyen et al. [56] and Wang et al. [57] in *Cajanus cajan, Secale cereale* L., *Zea mays* L. and *Triticum aestivum*.

8. Efficacy of soybean genetic manipulation

It has been more than two decades, since the introduction of genetically modified plants established through *in vitro Agrobacterium*-mediated transformation. In soybean, the first successful transformation was reported by Hinchee et al. [58], using cotyledonary explants with *Agrobacterium* pTiT37-SE harbouring pMON9749 for herbicide glyphosate tolerance. The success in this method depended upon several factors; which included tissue culture conditions, strains of *Agrobacterium* used and the selected host plant genotypes aimed at receiving the transgenes. To date, this technique has succeeded in the production of high yielding transgenic plants, particularly for corn, chickpea, rice, cowpea, as well as a few new soybean cultivars [59–62].

Genetic transformation is now considered the most economic and highly effective method of genetic engineering that has been reported so far. The method holds the potential and promise to efficiently regenerate transgenic plants, especially for recalcitrant legume crops. Legumes like soybeans are some of the most important pulse crops and a good source of high quality proteins and oils, required for human consumption, health benefits and industrial processing. However, the vegetative and reproductive stages of soybean continuously show high sensitivity to biotic and abiotic stress constraints. Yield quality and quantity of this crop is severely affected by high temperatures, chilling, waterlogging and water deficit stress [2]. Furthermore, tools such as genetic engineering, aimed at improving the growth characteristics of this crop are also negatively influenced by several factors like genotype specificity and co-cultivation challenges discussed in the above sections. To circumvent challenges posed by all stress factors; an efficient and rapid system of transformation that develops non-chimeric transgenic plants with resistance to these conditions must be advanced. A genetic transformation that eliminates the problem of genotype specificity in many established protocols must be established. This generally implies that, a protocol developed for one cultivar must be efficiently used for the genetic transformation of other varieties, including species closely related to the same genera.

9. Final considerations and benefits for developing countries

The findings presented in this study clearly indicate that, the induction of transformed callus tissues and regeneration of transgenic plantlets through cotyledonary node method of soybean transformation in tissue culture still present serious challenges. The study further highlighted poor plant tissue culture reproducibility, less culture efficiency and genotype specificity as some of the major obstacles. The lack of a stably routine transformation protocol for genetic manipulation of soybean will encourage transformation rates to remain at less than 10% efficiency. The lower transformation rates affect distribution of better transgenic cultivars availability for farmers, encourage the continued losses in yields and the deterioration of soy-products quality. This has a direct negative impact on the growth and well-being of many human lives, animals and countries' economy. Soybean could be a driving force behind the development of many economies, particularly in Africa. Country's growth and stability, food security and other United Nation related strategic goals will be achieved, if there is full commercial exploitation of benefits offered by important agro-economic crops such as soybean.

Genetic transformation is a tool that could guarantee continuous productivity of crops even under severe climatic conditions. Floods, chilling and drought are major causes of yield losses in many regions, particularly in developing countries. Crops like soybean, are considered major rainy season pulses [63] and their growth is highly sensitive to water-deficit stress. Introduction of soybean cultivars with improved traits will immensely benefit farmers, enhancing cropping intensity and increased profitability per unit land area as discussed by Agarwal et al. [63]. Soybean will continue to remain a major oilseed crop. Its potential use in industrial production of biodiesel, current pharmaceutical and nutritional uses still encourages improvement of modern and conventional breeding systems. The systems need to be improved in order to develop novel varieties that meet the current environmental challenges, raise yields to unprecedented levels and feed the world-wide increasing populations. Finally, the success in the development of new varieties will allow for the incorporation of soybeans in daily diet. In developing countries for example; South Africa, soybean is used mainly for the manufacturing of animal feeds and vegetable oil. Direct human consumption of soybean makes a very smaller portion of the population's diet as indicated by Dlamini et al. [64].

10. Recommended strategies for improvements

There is adequate evidence gathered in this study indicating that, the soybean genotypes used will variably express and transmit the transgenes if any event of transformation is to take place. This was clearly demonstrated by the varied responses formed in plant cell initiation and microshoots formation during callus induction and shoot multiplication. Moreover, the varied intensities in oxidative browning of tissues, chlorosis and subsequent wounded tissue necrosis exhibited by explant from different genotypes, indicated the extend of the problems associated with *Agrobacterium*-mediated genetic transformation of legumes. For the successful optimisation of protocol routinely used for transformation of a wide range of soybean varieties, this tool requires the following amendments:

1. Thorough screening and selection of genotypes such as Peking that showed moderate level of resistance to production of phenolics and subsequent oxidation of tissues.
2. Re-evaluation of culture condition, particularly the amount and type of antibiotics used in the culture medium. Mangena [29] reported successful induction of multiple shoots from cotyledonary-node explants infected with *Agrobacterium tumefaciens* containing ΩPKY vector construct on MS medium containing aminoglycoside antibiotics. This study reported effective *Agrobacterium* overgrowth control, low explant toxicity, lower levels of explant decay and better shoot proliferation under aminoglycosides compared to the β-lactam antibiotics at a range between 50 and 500 mgL^{-1}.
3. Continued and effective use of additives. Culture agents that inhibit tissue senescence which include, but not limited to cysteine, dithiothreitol, ascorbate and sodium thiosulfate are highly recommended. The effectively optimised use of these antioxidants may have given positive results in cultivars like Peking than in any of the cultivars used.
4. *Agrobacterium tumefaciens* density must be thoroughly adjusted and optimised to avoid tissue senescence. Explant infection by this bacterium on the cotyledonary junctions and bases of explants causes tissue decay in culture. This effect occurs even though contamination as a result of *Agrobacterium* overgrowth is efficiently controlled.

Other affordable method such as *in-planta Agro*-injection must be considered by laboratories to generate new genetically improved soybean plants. This technique was introduced by Chee et al. [65] in genetic transformation of soybean and kidney bean by *Agro*-injecting seeds with a suspension of *Agrobacterium* strain EHA101 with pIG121 vector plasmid containing genes for neomycin phosphotransferase (NPTII), hygromycin phosphotransferase (HPT) and β-glucuronidase (GUS). The soybean and kidney bean seeds were surface sterilised using 0.6% sodium hypochlorite and germinated on moistened sterile paper towels at 25°C for 24 h in darkness. *Agro*-infection yielded 12% transgenic soybeans and 24% of transgenic kidney beans identified using NPTII amplified by polymerase chain reaction (PCR). Generally, there are difficulties in the *in vitro* regeneration and selection of transgenic plants during *Agrobacterium*-mediated genetic transformation. But, this technique is undoubtedly the best tool available for the transfer and expression of transfer DNA in host plant cells.

11. Conclusions

The use of double cotyledonary-node explants still remain superior for establishment of soybean cultures–callus and shoot proliferation. This is so, because the efficiency of the cultures established relied primarily on the explant type, as one of the culture factors. Explant amenability to *Agrobacterium* infection, antibiotics and growth regulator regimes impacted highly on the culture successes observed. A successful shoot and callus induction in the control media was illustrated. The negative impacts of *Agrobacterium* infection and effect of antibiotics on the culture was also observed. However, these findings clearly demonstrate that, more work still need to done, focusing on the optimisation of tissue culture conditions and bacterial cultures. For the main purpose of developing a high frequency, genotype independent and efficient protocol for use in *Agrobacterium*-mediated genetic transformation of soybean.

Acknowledgements

I would like to sincerely acknowledge the financial support by the Department of Higher Education and Training (DHET), under the New Generation of Academics Programme (nGAP), South Africa.

Thanks

My sincere gratitude and thanks goes to Dr. P.W. Mokwala and Prof R.V. Nikolova for their support and mentorship. Their words of encouragement will continue ringing in my ears. Many thanks to my family, friends, colleagues and the entire Department of Biodiversity for their support.

Author details

Phetole Mangena

Address all correspondence to: mangena.phetole@gmail.com

Department of Biodiversity, School of Molecular and Life Sciences, University of Limpopo, Sovenga, South Africa

References

[1] Messina MJ. Legumes and soybeans: Overview of their nutritional profiles and health effects. American Society for Clinical Nutrition. 1999;**70**(3):439-450

[2] Mangena P, Mokwala PW, Nikolova RV. Challenges of *in vitro* and *in vivo Agrobacterium*-mediated genetic transformation in soybean. In: Kasai M, editor. Soybean: The Basis of Yield, Biomass and Productivity. InTech Open Science: 2017. p. 75-94

[3] Sinclair TR, Marrou H, Soltani A, Vadez V, Chandolu KC. Soybean production potential in Africa. Global Food Security. 2014;**3**(1):31-40

[4] Kado C. Grown gall tumors. In: Brenner S, Miller JH, editors. Encyclopedia of Genetics. USA: Academic Press; 2001. pp. 491-393

[5] Tefera H. Breeding for promiscuous soybeans at IITA. In: Sudaric A, editor. Soybean-Molecular Aspects of Breeding. Croatia: InTech Open Science; 2011. p. 147-162

[6] Hinchee MAM, Connor-Ward DV, Newell CA, McConnell RE, Sato SJ, Gasser CS, Fischhoff DA, Re DB, Fraley RT, Horsch RB. Production of transgenic soybean plants using Agrobacterium-mediated DNA transfer. Biotechnology Journal. 1988;**6**:915-922

[7] Vucenik I, Yang GY, Shamsuddin AM. Comparison of pure inositol hexaphosphate and high-bran diet in the prevention of DMBA-induced rat mammary carcinogenesis. Nutrition and Cancer. 1997;**28**:7-13

[8] Hunt JR, Gallagher SK, Johnson LK. Effect of ascorbic acid on apparent ion absorption by women with low iron stores. American Journal of Clinical Nutrition. 1994;**59**:1381-1385

[9] Daly LE, Kirke PN, Molloy A, Weir DG, Scott JM. Folate levels and neural tube defects. Journal of the American Medical Association. 1995;**274**:1698-1702

[10] Du Plessis M. Cysteine proteases activity and gene expression studies in soybean nodules during development and drought stress [Master's dissertation]. South Africa: University of Pretoria; 2013

[11] Beers EP, Woffenden BJ, Zhao C. Plant proteolytic enzymes: Possible roles during programmed cell death. Plant Molecular Biology. 2000;**44**:399-415

[12] Ishida Y, Saito H, Ohta S, Hiei Y, Komari T, Kumashiro T. High efficiency transformation of maize (*Zea mays* L.) mediated by *Agrobacterium tumefaciens*. Nature Biotechnology. 1996; **14**:745-750

[13] Popelka JC, Gollasch S, Moore A, Molvig L, Higgins TJV. Genetic transformation of transgenes to progeny. Plant Cell Reports. 2006;**25**(4):304-312

[14] Rao KS, Rohini VK, *Agrobacterium*-mediated transformation of sunflower (*Helianthus annuus* L.): A simple protocol. Annals of Botany 1999;**83**:347-354

[15] Cardoza V, Stewart Jr CN. Agrobacterium-mediated transformation of Canola. In: Curtis IS, editor. Transgenic Crops of the World: Essential Protocols. Netherlands: Kluwer Academic Publishers; 2004. p. 379-387

[16] Ashikari M, Matsuoka M, Datta Sk. Transgenic rice plants. In: Curtis IS, editor. Transgenic Crops of the World: Essential Protocols. Netherlands: Kluwer Academic Publishers; 2004. p. 3-18

[17] Christie PJ, Gordon JE. The *Agrobacterium* Ti plasmids. Microbiology Spectrum. 2014; **2**(6):1-29

[18] Finer J, Dhillon T. Transgenic plant production. In: Stewart CN Jr, editor. Plant Biotechnology and Genetics: Principles, Techniques and Applications. New Jersey: Wiley; 2008. 246 p

[19] Vaucheret H. Promoter-dependent trans-inactivation in transgenic tobacco plants: Kinetic aspects of gene silencing and gene reactivation. Comptes Rendus de l'Académie des Sciences. Series III. 1994;**317**:310-323

[20] Zhao H, Tan Z, Wen X, Wang Y. An improved syringe agroinfiltration protocol to enhance transformation efficiency by combinative use if 5-azacytidine, ascorbate acid and Tween-20. Plants. 2017;**6**(9):1-10

[21] Verma SS, Chinnusamy V, Bansa KC. A simplified floral dip method for transformation of *Brassica napus* and *B. carinata*. Journal of Plant Biochemistry and Biotechnology. 2008;**17**(2):197-200

[22] Kikkert JR, Vidal JR, Reisch BI. Stable transformation of plant cells by particle bombardment/biolistics. Methods in Molecular Biology. 2005;**286**:61-78

[23] Zia M. Soybean: Plant manipulation to Agrobacterium mediated transformation. In: Krezhowa D, editor. Soybean- Genetics and Novel Techniques for Yield Enhancement. Croatia: In Tech Open Science; 2011. p. 297-310

[24] Shou H, Frame BR, Whitham SA, Wang K. Assessment of transgenic maize events produced by particle bombardment or *Agrobacterium*-mediated transformation. Molecular Breeding. 2004;**13**:201-208

[25] Karami O. Factors affecting *Agrobacterium*-mediated transformation of plants. Transgenic Plant Journal. 2008;**2**(2):127-137

[26] Mangena P, Mokwala PW, Nikolova RV. Challenges of *in vitro* and *in vivo* Agrobacterium-mediated genetic transformation in soybean. In: Kasai M, editor. Soybean: The Basis of Yield, Biomass and Productivity. Croatia: InTech Open Science; 2017. p. 75-94

[27] Zhang L, Yang XD, Zhang Y, Yang J, Qi G, Guo D, Xing G, Yao Y, Xu W, Li H, Li Q, Dong D. Changes in oleic acid content of transgenic soybeans by antisense RNA mediated post-transcriptional gene silencing. International Journal of Genomics. 2014:1-8

[28] Raza G, Singh MB, Bhalla PL. *In vitro* plant regeneration from commercial cultivars of soybean. BioMed Research International. 2017:1-9

[29] Mangena P. Oryza cystatin 1 based genetic transformation in soybean for drought tolerance [Masters dissertation]. South Africa: University of Limpopo; 2015

[30] Heatherly LG. Drought stress and irrigation effects on germination of harvested soybean seed. Crop Science. 1993;**22**(4):777-781

[31] Desclaux D, Hugnh TT, Roumet P. Identification of soybean plant characteristics that indicate the timing of drought stress. Crop Science. 2000;**40**(3):716-722

[32] Brown E, Brown D, Caviness C. Response of selected soybean cultivar to soil moisture deficit. Agronomy Journal. 1985;**77**(2):274-278

[33] Singh J, Singh D. Biodiesel production through the use of different sources and characterization of oil and their esters as the substitute of diesel: A review. Renewable and Sustainable Energy Review. 2010;**41**(1):200-216

[34] Mielenz JR, Bardsley JS, Wyman CE. Fermentation of soybean hulls to ethanol while preserving protein value. Bioresource Technology. 2009;**14**:3532-3539

[35] Yu Y, Liang H, Wang S, Lian Y, Wei Y, Wang T. Research progress and commercialization on transgenic soybean in China. Soybean Science. 2010;**29**:143-150

[36] Pierik RLM. *In Vitro* Culture of Higher Plants. United Kingdom: Martinus Mishoff Publishers; 1997. pp. 89-100

[37] Paz MM, Martinez JC, Kalvig AB, Fonger TM, Wang K. Improved cotyledonary-node method using an alternative explant derived from mature seed for efficient *Agrobacterium*-mediate soybean transformation. Plant Cell Reports. 2006;**25**:206-213

[38] Mangena P, Mokwala PW, Nikolova RV. *In vitro* multiple shoot induction in soybean. International Journal of Agriculture and Biology. 2015;**17**:838-842

[39] El-Kaaby EA, Al-Hattab ZN, Al-Anny JA. FT-IR identification of capsaicin from callus and seedling of chilli pepper plants *Capsicum annuum* L. *in vitro*. International Journal of Multidisciplinary and Current Research. 2016;**4**:1144-1146

[40] Bahry CA, Perboni AT, Nardino M, Zimmer PD. Physiological quality and inhibitions of soybean seeds with contrasting coats. Revista Ciência Agronômica. 2017;**48**(1):125-133

[41] Zhang BH, Liu F, Liu ZH, Wang HM, Yao CB. Effect of kanamycin on tissue culture and somatic embryogenesis in cotton. Plant Growth Regulation. 2001;**33**(2):137-149

[42] Grzebelus E, Skop L. Effect of β-lactam antibiotics on plant regeneration in carrot protoplast cultures. *In Vitro* Cellular Development and Biology–Plant. 2014;**50**(5):568-575

[43] Barwale UB, Kerns HR, Widholm JM. Plant regeneration from callus cultures of several soybean genotypes via embryogenesis and organogenesis. Planta. 1986;**167**:473-481

[44] Franklin CI, Dixon RA. Initiation and maintenance of callus and cell suspension cultures. In: Dixon RA, Gonzales RA, editors. Plant Cell Culture: A Practical Approach. 2nd ed. United Kingdom: Oxford University Press; 1995. pp. 16-21

[45] Yu TA, Yeh SD, Yang JS. Effect of carbenicillin and cefotaxime on callus growth and somatic embryogenesis from adventitious roots of papaya. Botanical Bulletin- Academia Sinica. 2001;**42**:281-286

[46] El-Siddig MA, El-Hussein AA, Siddig MAM, Elballa MMA, Saker MM. *Agrobacterium*-mediated transformation and *in-vitro* regeneration of tomato (*Lycopersicon esculentum* Mill) plants cv. Castlerock. Journal of Genetic Engineering and Biotechnology. 2009;**7**(1):11-17

[47] Yan B, Reddy MSS, Collins GB, Dinkins RD. *Agrobacterium*-mediated transformation of soybean [*Glycine max* (L.) Merrill] using immature zygotic cotyledon explants. Plant Cell Reports. 2000;**19**:1090-1097

[48] AMP J, Saxena PX. Inhibition of phenylpropanoid biosynthesis in *Artemisia annua* L.: A novel approach in reducing oxidative browning in plant tissue culture. PLoS One. 2013;**8**(10):e76802

[49] Li S, Cong Y, Liu Y, Wang T, Shuai Q, Chen N, Gai J, Li Y. Optimisation of *Agrobacterium*-mediated transformation in soybean. Frontiers in Plant Science. 2017;**8**(246):1-15

[50] Hartmann HT, Kester DE, Davies FT, Geneve RL. Hartmann and Kester's Plant Propagation: Principles and Practice. 8th ed. New Jersey: Prentice Hall; 2013. pp. 670-679

[51] Zhang Z, Xing A, Staswick P, Clemente TE. The use of glufosinate as a selective agent in *Agrobacterium*-mediated transformation of soybean. Plant Cell, Tissue and Organ Culture. 1999;**56**:37-46

[52] Paz MM, Huixia S, Zibiao G, Zhang Z, Anjan KB, Wang K. Assessment of conditions affecting *Agrobacterium*-mediated soybean transformation using the cotyledonary node explants. Plant Science. 2004;**136**:167-179

[53] Trolinder NL, Xhixian C. Genotype specificity of the somatic embryogenesis response in cotton. Plant Cell Reports. 1989;**8**:133-136

[54] Gawali PM, Akhare AA, Gahukar SJ. Genotype specificity for *in vitro* regenerability of pigeonpea genotypes. Asian Sciences. 2010;**51**(1):53-56

[55] Targonska M, Hromada-Judycka A, Bolibok-Bragoszewska H, Rakoczy-Trojanowska M. The specificity and genetic background of the rye (*Secale cereale* L.) tissue culture response. Plant Cell Reports. 2013;**32**(1):1-9

[56] Nguyen TN, Tran TL, Nguyen DT. *Agrobacterium*-mediated transformation of five inbred maize with the brittle 2 gene. Turkish Journal of Biodiversity. 2016;**40**:755-761

[57] Wang K, Liu H, Du L, Ye X. Generation of marker-free transgenic hexaploidy wheat via a *Agrobacterium*-mediated co-transformation strategy in commercial Chinese wheat varieties. Plant Biotechnology Journal. 2017;**15**:614-623

[58] Hinchee MAW, Connor-Ward DV, Newell CA, McDonnell RE, Sato SJ, Gasser CS, Fischhoff DA, Re DB, Fraley RT, Horsch RB. Production of transgenic soybean plants using *Agrobacterium*-mediated DNA transfer. Nature Biotechnology. 1988;**6**:915-922

[59] Ko TS, Nelson RL, Korban S. Screening multiple soybean cultivars (MG00 to MG VIII) for somatic embryogenesis following *Agrobacterium*-mediated transformation of immature cotyledons. Crop Science; **2004**(44):1825-1831

[60] Raveendar S, Ignacimuthu S. Improved *Agrobacterium*-mediated transformation in cowpea *Vigna unguiculata* L Walp. Asian Journal of Plant Sciences. 2010;**9**:256-263

[61] Mehrotra M, Sanyal I, Amla DV. High-efficiency *Agrobacterium*-mediated transformation of chickpea (*Cicer arietinum* L.) and regeneration of insect-resistant transgenic plants. Plant Cell Reports. 2011;**30**(9):1603-1616

[62] Patel M, Dewey RE, Qu R. Enhancing *Agrobacterium tumefaciens*-mediated transformation efficiency of perennial ryegrass and rice using heat and high maltose treatment during bacterial infection. Plant Cell Tissue and Organ Culture. 2013;**114**:19-29

[63] Agarwal DK, Billore SD, Sharma AN, Dupare BV, Srivastava SK. Soybean: Introduction, improvement and utilisation in India–Problems and prospects. Agricultural Research. 2013;**2**(4):293-300

[64] Dlamini TS, Tshabalala P, Mutengwa T. Soybeans production in South Africa. Oilseeds & Fats Crops and Lipids. 2014;**21**(2):1-11

[65] Chee PP, Goldman SL, Graves ACF, Slighton JL. Transformation of soybean (*Glycine max*) by infecting germinating seeds with *Agrobacterium* tumefaciens. Plant Physiology. 1989;**91**:1212-1218

Chapter 3

Understanding CRISPR/Cas9: A Magnificent Tool for Plant Genome Editing

Jorge Ricaño-Rodríguez, Jorge Suárez-Medellin, Eliezer Cocoletzi Vásquez, José M. Ramos-Prado and Enrique Hipólito-Romero

Additional information is available at the end of the chapter

http://dx.doi.org/10.5772/intechopen.81080

Abstract

Nowadays, it is well known that archaea organisms as well as bacteria show an important range of defense mechanisms. Among others, a unique molecular system called CRISPR/Cas (clustered regularly interspaced short palindromic repeats) helps provide protection (adaptive guided immunity) athwart foreign nucleic acids, including plasmids and viral infections. As a typical immune response, CRISPR system is based on the acquisition of genetic records provided by infectious external agents, and in this sense, a high interference upon a new infection is unchained. In relation to plant research, less than 10 years ago, efforts to understand this peculiar mechanism and the possibility of being used in biotechnological processes have been focused on obtaining atavistic changes in different transformable vegetal specimens by inducing selective mutations into a reading frame that may be translated in a given moment (i.e., ORF; open reading frame). In light of the consideration that one common use of ORFs is to assist gene prediction processes, palindromic repeats are mostly based on the directed mutations via nonhomologous end joining. Although it is true that DNA-free editing techniques are now desirable for molecular crop breeding, CRISPR/Cas as a mutational regulatory system in plant biology may offer better complex genome rearrangements.

Keywords: CRISPR/Cas9, plant genome editing, molecular crop breeding, RNA guided DNA, Cas9 nuclease

1. Introduction

Sustainable agriculture is considered to be the key for improving plant crops through genetic engineering, since random mutagenesis processes are part of conventional biotechnology techniques used for most researchers in this field [1]. CRISPR/Cas9 systems (clustered regularly interspaced short palindromic repeats-CRISPR associated) are related to a well-known CRISPR array defined by series of 20–50 bp genomic locus (i.e., unique spacers separated by direct repeats).

On the other hand, these unique spacers usually have similar length with preceded AT-rich fragments [2]. CRISPR loci were identified for the first time about two decades ago when they found a series of short genomic sequences (i.e., spacers) in *Escherichia coli* originated by viral genomes and probably due to the presence of conjugative plasmids, and in this sense, the foreign genetic material allowed the bacteria to record a kind of memory (e.g., immune system) to counteract future infections. When foreign DNA sequences match these unique spacers, they are commonly known as "photospacers" [1, 3]. Thereby, the corresponding immunization is against a foreign phage (e.g.), and when a new infection of this nature takes place in the future, the array expansion of the CRISPR is unchained and in consequence, new spacers originate from the genetic material of the phage.

According to some authors [4–6], this interesting immune system (to call it that) may be divided into three metabolic stages: adaptation, crRNA (CRISPR-RNAs) biogenesis, and interference. When a foreign DNA introduction happens, there is a selective process through the machinery that selects protospacers, which will be inserted into the CRISPR locus (insertion takes place into the leader end of the system). In the first stage of crRNA biogenesis, a transcription of CRISPR locus is observed followed by a direct processing of sequence elements (pre-crRNAs–crRNAs), all of them with the corresponding single spacer. After this stage, Cas proteins interact the crRNAs by assembling an effector complex (**Figure 1A**) [4]. This is very important since these components are intermediary elements of the interference stage where recognition of foreign DNA happens upon future infections and consequently, its degradation. It is very important to mention that a spacer acquisition creates genetic records of previous infections; as mentioned above, CRISPR immunity happens when there is an imminent detection of strange nucleic acids and consequently, the integration of foreign genetic material into the host's cells (the DNA integration occurs in the chromosome).

CRISPR systems are highly complex and diverse, and nowadays, efforts have been made to classify them into six interesting types: Type I (eight different Cas representative operons); Type II (tracrRNA; trans-activating crRNA and four Cas); Type III (eight Cas and Csm/Cmr); Type IV (four DinG/Csf); Type V (four Cas/Cpf2); and Type VI (three Cas/C2c2). In this case, operon type IV shows an extensive presence in the lack of CRISPR loci (**Figure 1B**) [4].

Due to the endless background that precede the functionality and applications of CRISPR systems in the field of genetic engineering, it has been shown that this metabolic phenomenon is extremely attractive for the molecularly directed crop improvement as well as plant genomic research. In general, the efforts that outline research for CRISPR systems within the agronomic

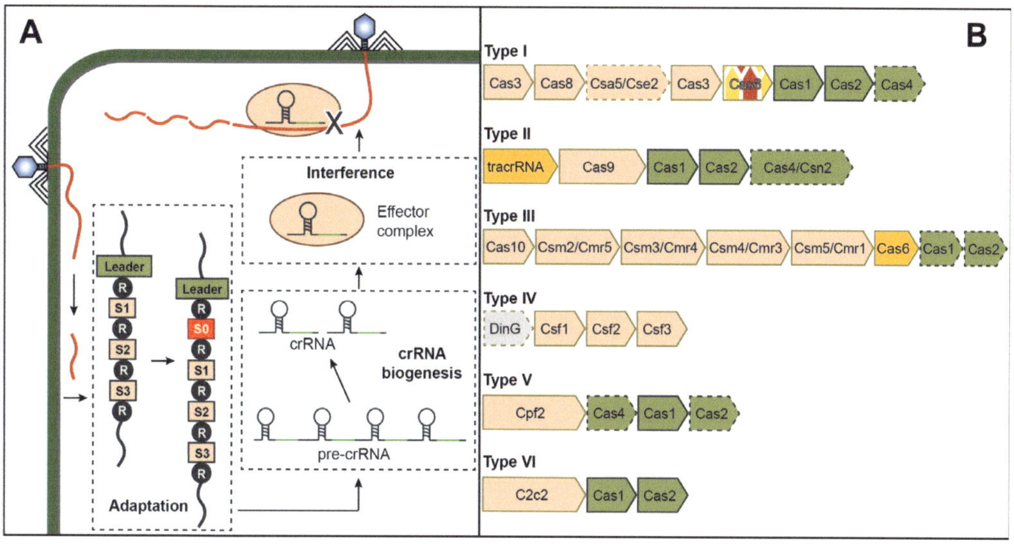

Figure 1. Functional and organizational system of the CRISPR/Cas9. (A) The process of induced immunity is carried out in three stages consisting of an adaptation, crRNA biogenesis, and interference. In the first stage, the adaptive machinery performs a selection of photospacers, and they are leader-end inserted into CRISPR locus that is subsequently transcribed during crRNA biogenesis. In a complementary way, the pre-crRNA processing into crRNAs with simple spacers is developed. Finally, the effector complex is originated through the assembly of crRNA with Cas proteins, which interacts (interference stage) in a subsequent way to the infection, and consequent degradation of the foreign genetic material. (B) Structurally, the CRISPR system is divided into six representative types (operons). Dashed outlines represent genes in some subtypes. Pink sequences represent genes related to the interference process. Yellow sequences refer to crRNA biogenesis, and the green color refers to adaptation genes. Subtypes IV are characterized by the absence of CRISPR loci. Adapted from Wright et al. [4].

sciences field have been mainly focused on plant domestication with economic and social interest. Thus, interspaced short palindromic repeats constantly open the doors to the generation and knowledge application in the area of functional genomics that jointly guide researchers toward the implementation of theoretical and applied biostrategies [7].

2. CRISPR/Cas9 mechanism: brief overview of its nature

The action mode of CRISPR/Cas9 biological system is basically based on the participation of two distinct elements: the Cas9 protein (CRISPR-associated protein 9; RNA-guided DNA endonuclease enzyme associated with CRISPR) and sgRNA (single guide RNA) [8]. Nowadays, Cas9 proteins are found mainly in different bacteria species such as *Brevibacillus laterosporus* [9], *Staphylococcus aureus* [10], and other representative species within the genus *Streptococcus* [11]. Cas9 proteins have shown two representative domains: the first one is known as HNH (nuclease-associated proteins), which is responsible for cleaving and regrouping the complementary strand of crRNA. On the other hand, the second domain known as RuvC-like (nuclease domain that cleaves complementary DNA strands) has the purpose of carrying out the cleavage of the complementary strand of dsDNA (double stranded

DNA). The nature of the sgRNA is extremely curious, since this is a kind of synthetic RNA with a length not greater than 100 bp and whose structure owns a 20 bp sequence coupled to the 5′-end that works as a guide allowing the identification of target sequences through specific adjacent motifs (i.e., PAM sequences; protospacer adjacent motifs) [8].

It is important to mention that 3′-end of the sgRNA resembles a loop structure that allows it to develop a very precise linkage with the target sequence. This is the way to structure a new complex that will be associated with Cas9 and in this sense, to perform the dsDNA cleavage that will cause double-stranded breaks (DSBs) [12]. Generally, a DSB is the result of the continuous DNA damage at chromosome level, although this is considered a completely normal phenomenon within the cell. However, the resulting by-products generated by the cellular metabolism itself such as reactive oxygen species (ROS) may interfere in the replication process due to the damage caused in the DNA. Also, environmental selective pressures as different chemical agents or UV light itself are considered other important factors involved in this process [13, 14].

When the above phenomenon has been carried out within the cell, the presence of DSBs activates the repair mechanism of damaged DNA through nonhomologous end joining (NHEJ) or homology-directed repair (HDR). In most cases, the repair of DBSs is carried out by NHEJ although the main reason why this happens is because it is the best way to make genetic insertions or deletions and consequently to give rise to a gene knockout (gene knockout is a genetic phenomenon through which an organism's gene becomes inoperative). In general, HDR is originated by the presence of an oligo template, and it activates the elimination of specific genes as well as foreign DNA (the mechanism involves the substitution of DNA sequences in a specific locus, or well, fragment sequences not found within this locus) [8, 12–15]. In addition to CRISPR, there are other methods currently used for genome editing which include the participation of peculiar endonucleases such as transcription activator-link effectors (TALEN) and zinc fingers. Through these mechanisms, a fusion between DNA-binding domains of transcription factors and the nuclease domain FokI (restriction enzyme) takes place. Beyond the application of CRISPR systems in genome editing and their regulation processes, these types of endonucleases may be used to be fused with fluorescent proteins in order to allow more specific loci location within the living cells [16, 17].

3. Cas9 enzyme: multifunctional DNA endonuclease

The Cas9 enzyme has a very peculiar structure since it consists of two distinct nodes complemented each other: an alpha-helical recognition site (REC) and an endonuclease structure (NUC) containing HNH proteins. On the other hand, Cas9 structure has RuvC-like and C-terminal domains with variable structures [18]. Both nodes are linked through anchoring-like structures mostly conformed by arginine-rich bridges and other less complex structures generally observed between residues 712–720. In this sense, there are three very important domains with alpha-helical structure that integrate the REC node (Hel-I, II, and III) and as an interesting fact; Hel domains show no structural similarity with some other known proteins to date [19].

Several studies have shown that Cas9/RuvC domains have very similar structures to retroviral integrases (virally encoded; specialized recombinases capable of catalyzing the recombination of viral DNA particles into the genome's host cell). In contrast to the above, the HNH nuclease domains show a fold-type $\beta\beta\alpha$ structure linked to a metallic cofactor that in the same way, it is linked to another HNH domain from a different endonuclease that allows the recognition through metallic ions in order to locate cleavage sites on the target DNA sequence [18]. Metallic ion-dependent restriction enzymes show highly conserved structures formed by aspartate residues and in less quantity by histidine [20].

In basal conditions, the nature of Cas9 enables the enzyme to be inactive and when a recombination between sgRNA and the corresponding REC lobe is observed, it is precisely that this natural state changes. Thus, the previous complex performs a specific search for PAMs (trinucleotide NGG) in order to identify target sequences into the double DNA strand. When a linkage has happened within the respective PAMPS, a cleavage of the hybrid DNA-RNA complex takes place thanks to HNH domain and, jointly, RuvC assists the structuring of dsSDBs (double-stranded SDBs) by cleaving the corresponding complementary sequence [21]. It is important to mention that both eukaryotic and prokaryotic cells show NHEJ and HDR mechanisms capable of repairing DSBs through the intervention of DNA ligase IV, whose nature helps regroup damaged nucleotide ends (Indels; introduction or deletion of mutations) as well as the use of complementary homologous DNA templates, respectively [21, 22].

Within the group of Cas9 proteins, there are repression effectors that are fused with a transcription activation system called dCas9 (CRISPR tool based on a modified version of the Cas9 protein). The dCas9 systems are usually combined with effector protein domains that regroup functional peptides that will target specific regions of genome loci. Thus, the resulting complex performs activation and shutdown mechanisms of gene repression, thereby; it is considered an efficient regulator of genetic information flow. This is why CRISPR/dCas9 system may be a modular platform in several cellular processes to control transcription [21, 23]. Another important fact about the dCas9 complexes is that they are able to combine with different epigenetic nature molecules, such as methylation and histone peptides [24].

On the other hand, specificity is a considerable element in genome editing tools. In the case of Cas9/gRNA (guide RNA) complexes, they have an extremely precise capacity to develop cleavages in DNA sequences, even when small mismatches may be observed into the guide template [25]. When this type of phenomenon happens, nonspecific cleavages are mostly tolerated at the 5′-ends or at a greater distance from the corresponding MAMP sequences. It has been noticed that short gRNAs (a.c. 20 bp) confer better specificity to Cas9 proteins at the target cleavage sites within the genetic editing processes [26]. Likewise, when the inactivation of Cas9 conserved domains is observed, a specific break occurs in one of the DNA strands (nickase), which leads to a splitting and loss of its double-stranded native structure [27]. In general, this type of nicks usually causes no mutations since they can be repaired in a very simple way by eliminating damaged bases through a specific repair metabolic pathway.

4. CRISPR/Cas9: a close relationship with TALENs and ZFNs

As previously mentioned, CRISPR/Cas9 system is conformed by a single monomeric protein as well as a complex RNA rearrangement. The Cas9 protein is responsible for carrying out the cleavage process, and a 20-nt fragment corresponding to gRNA is responsible for identifying target sequences [28]. Notwithstanding, the nature of TALENs and ZFNs (zinc finger nucleases) allows them to function as dimers; consequently, protein components are just required to develop the corresponding catalysis processes. A specific domain of the FokI endonuclease performs the cleavage of target sequences. On the other hand, domains corresponding to DNA binding that may be found in different polypeptides are those that confer the sequence specificity [29].

Because ZFNs show a necessary interaction with zinc fingers, it is considered that this process is experimentally complicated, and therefore, its application is usually limited within a biotechnological context, especially considering the need for nucleotide sequence specificity. However, TALENs and ZFNs are easy to design, and they are commercially available in most cases at an affordable cost [30]. TALENs can promote homologous recombination at cellular level through repetitive sequences compared to gRNA that is based on a Watson-Crick baseparing principle using target DNA sequences [28, 30]. On the other hand, TALENs and ZFNs are capable of generating DSBs through the restriction of FokI catalytic domains of different overlap sizes that may vary depending on their binding capacity. In comparison, Cas9 has two cleavage domains as previously discussed (i.e., RuvC and HNH). While it is true that ZFNs could target any sequence of interest, this process is subject to the availability of assembly platforms. Today, available molecular libraries can hold up to 100 bp sequences that serve as platforms for functional ZFNs. Thereby, TALEN's targets require thymidine residues to show an efficient functionality, which could limit their application [31].

TALEN protein arrays are exclusive for the group of plant pathogenic bacteria. The repeated sequences comprise 10–20 residue agglomerates that recognize specific DNA molecules. Each repeat has a maximum of 35 amino acids in length, and it is complemented by two adjacent amino acids (RVD, repeat-variable-di-residue) which have the function of conferring specificity to the four nucleotides that structure the DNA strands. In this way, a direct link between repeated sequences and target DNA is observed. Both TALENs and ZFNs are capable of generating DSBs in a specific region of the genome, and as previously discussed, this phenomenon is commonly used to generate gene knock out. RVD codes are used to generate TALEN repeating arrays, and therefore, an affinity of up to 96% can be observed respect to target sequences of interest [31, 32]. It is worth mentioning that TALENs show advantages over ZFNs, for example, TALENs can be extended over any sequence length that is necessary, and for the case of ZFNs, they can only be extended in a range of 9–18 bp, although it is considered that TALENs show less specificity [33].

A disadvantage of TALENs over ZFNs is their considerable size, since the extension of a cDNA sequence encoded by TALENs can be up to 3 kb, while the size per every ZFN is only 1 kb. The considerable size of TALENs could hinder the recombination process at cellular level, and therefore, these arrangements tend to be less attractive for biotechnological processes, mainly in therapeutic applications. On the other hand, since TALENs show repetitive nature, it is usually more complicated to pack and move the molecules into the host cell using viral vectors [31].

In the case of ZFNs, it is important to highlight that in recent years, their use has increased considerably in both industrial and basic research, mainly for the generation of therapeutic adjuvants in both animal and human models. ZFNs comprise arrays of protein fusions with specific binding domains adapted to transcription factors that contain zinc finger complements. In a complementary way, its structure is also conformed by a FokI restriction domain. The zinc finger domains are able to recognize 3–4 bp sequences in the target DNA molecule. Tandem domains (tandem repeats; occurring in the DNA through the repetition of patterns of one or more nucleotides and the position of these is completely adjacent) tend to interlace with nucleotide sequences between 3, 9, and 18 bp length, and this process is repetitive throughout

Species	Cas9 codon	Trans method	Target sequence	Promoter	Mutation rate	Detection method	Ref
Arabidopsis thaliana	*Arabidopsis* (intron)	PEG protoplast	PDS3, FLS2	CaMV35SPDK, AtU6	1.1–5.6%	PCR sequencing	[36]
A. thaliana	*Arabidopsis* (intron)	PEG protoplast	RACK1b, RACK1c	CaMV35SPDK, AtU6	2.5–2.7%	PCR sequencing	[36]
Nicotiana benthamiana	*Arabidopsis* (intron)	PEG protoplast	PDS3	CaMV35SPDK, AtU6	37.7–38.5%	PCR sequencing	[36]
N. benthamiana	*Chlamydomonas reinhardtii*	Leaf agroinfiltration	Co-transfect GFP	CaMV35S, AtU6	n.a.	Pre-digested PCR	[37, 38]
N. benthamiana	Human	Leaf agroinfiltration	PDS	CaMV35S, CaMV35S	12.7–13.8%	n.a.	[39]
Oryza sativa	Rice	PEG protoplast	PDS, BADH2, MPK2, Os02g2382	2xCaMV35S, OsU3	14.5–38%	PCR	[40]
O. sativa	Human	PEG protoplast	MPK5	CaMV35S, OsU3 or OsU6	3–8%	qPCR and T7E1 assay	[14]
O. sativa	Rice	PEG protoplast	SWEET14	CaMV35S, OsU6	n.a.	Pre-digested PCR	[37, 38]
Triticum aestivum	Rice	PEG protoplast	MLO	2xCaMV35S, TaU6	28.5%	PCR + RE	[40]
T. aestivum	Human	Agro-transfect embryo immature cell	PDS, INOX	CaMV35S	18–22%	PCR sequencing	[39]
Zea mays	Rice	PEG protoplast	IPK	2xCaMV35S, ZmU3	16.4–19.1%	n.a.	[41]
Citrus sinensis	Human	Leaf agro-infiltration	PDS	CaMv35S, CaMV35S	3.2–3.9%	PCR + RE	[42]

Table 1. Examples of plant transient transfection based on CRISPR/Cas9-mediated NHEJ.

the entire genome in question. ZFNs act at two sites of the DNA sequence at the cellular level, on the forward and reverse strand, respectively. Since cleavages of specific regions within the genome can be observed, ZFNs are capable to recognize two adjacent sequences, and once the corresponding cleavage occurs, the FokI restriction enzyme domains produce a dimerization prior to the cleavage of the corresponding DNA loci. Thus, DSBs with 5′-extensions originate [31, 34, 35]. As listed in **Table 1**, some examples of experiments related to transient transfection based on CRISPR/Cas9-mediated NHEJ may be cited.

5. CRISPR/Cas9 applications in crop genetic improvement: brief overview

The relevance of agriculture for human survival is hard to underestimate. Crops provide food, fiber, and raw materials for a growing human population that faces an increasing amount of challenges, including loss and degradation of arable land as well as climate change. In this context, the rational use of all the available biotechnological tools is of paramount importance to attain a worthy life quality both in developed countries and the third world. Crop genome editing is among the most promising techniques to cope with the aforementioned agricultural challenges. However, it is worth noting that the development of those methodologies is useful not only for genetic improvement of agricultural crops but also to functional characterization of specific plant genes for basic research purposes [43].

Three short reports, published in 2013, demonstrated the feasibility of CRISPR/Cas9 system for genetic engineering of crops, based on the pioneer works of Li et al. (using *A. thaliana*), Nekrasov et al. (with *N. benthamiana*), and Shan et al. (*O. sativa* and *T. aestivum*), respectively [36, 40, 44]. After that, a plethora of research on crop genome editing has been published. The works listed below include some of the most representative studies on the matter, according to our best knowledge. However, the amazing dynamism of the field makes the presumption of exhaustiveness unattainable.

Given its undeniable worldwide relevance as a staple food, it is not surprising that rice has been one of the most studied crops in terms of CRISPR/Cas9 mediated genetic edition [14, 38, 45–48]. Among the main modifications proposed to this crop, it can be found herbicide resistance [49, 50], improved nitrogen use efficiency [51], and resistance against the rice blast disease [52].

Wheat (both durum and bread wheat) has also been subjected to extensive research in order to optimize the effectiveness of the genome editing process [53–55] as well as the acquisition of novel attributes including heritable broad-spectrum resistance to powdery mildew and other plant diseases [56].

Other crops widely used for the validation of technical improvements in CRISPR/Cas9 system are soybean [12, 57, 58] and maize [59, 60]. The latter cereal has also been modified in order to exhibit advantageous traits. For instance, this technology has generated novel variants of the ARGOS8 gene on maize. The ARGOS8 edited variants significantly increased grain yield under drought stress conditions, compared to wild-type maize, and had no yield loss under normal conditions [61].

The CRISPR/Cas9 system was also used to investigate the influence of specific genes on the phenotype development in tomato plants [51, 62, 63], as well as to achieve features of agronomic importance, such as delayed ripening of tomato fruit [64] or parthenocarpy [65]. Other members of the *Solanaceae* family reported to have undergone genetic editing via CRISPR/Cas9, include tobacco (*Nicotiana tabacum*) [38, 66], potato (*Solanum tuberosum*) [67], and petunia (*Petunia hybrida*) [68].

The CRISPR/Cas9 technology has also been used to confer molecular immunity against tomato yellow leaf curl virus (TYLCV), using *N. benthamiana* as host [69], as well as inducing complete resistance to Turnip mosaic virus (TuMV) [70], and improve the stress response in the model plant *A. thaliana* [71].

In the case of the emerging oil seed plant, *Camelina sativa*, the CRISPR/Cas9-targeted genetic edition has improved its fatty acid composition, obtaining a seed oil of superior quality on multiple levels, which besides being healthier, was more stable to oxidation and better suited for biofuel production [72, 73].

In addition to that, this technology has been used to obtain a nontransgenic cucumber strain (*Cucumis sativus* L.), resistant to cucumber vein yellowing disease, papaya ringspot mosaic virus-W, and zucchini yellow mosaic virus [74], as well as to successfully induce targeted mutagenesis in the Chardonnay grape cultivar that enhanced its endurance to powdery mildew, and to increase the golden delicious apple cultivar resistance to fire blight disease [75].

Besides the aforementioned, other crops in which the CRISPR/Cas9 technology has been optimized include barley (*Hordeum vulgare*) and *Brassica oleracea* [76], watermelon (*Citrullus lanatus*) [77], as well as the nonherbaceous sweet orange (*C. sinensis* cultivar *Valencia*) [42] and poplar (*Populus tomentosa*) [78].

Finally, we would like to stress that there is no scientific evidence whatsoever to assume that genetic modifications produced by modern biotechnological tools, such as CRISPR/Cas9, represent a higher health or environmental risk than conventional breeding techniques. However, public distrust caused by genetically modified crops has led to many countries to implement highly strict and costly regulations that make very difficult to successfully commercialize such products. Interestingly, since CRISPR/Cas9 genetic editing does not necessarily implies the incorporation of foreign DNA, according to some interpretations, the existing legislation might not be applicable to this technology. Therefore, the scientifically informed public discussion of such legal framework is imperative [43, 75, 79].

6. Conclusions and final considerations

In recent years, the progress in the development of new tools for molecular genetic research has been evident since their application by simple, versatile, and efficient experimental techniques. From all the genome edition systems based on the nucleases application, CRISPR/Cas9 is the most friendly and simple method. It is now clear that the utility of this technology for the modification of specific loci is limited only by the interest of the researcher. In coming years, debates are expected about the best use of organic and conventional agriculture, sustainable farming, and all that coming from biotechnology. Thus, CRISPR/Cas9 technology has changed the way we see the future of agriculture. On the other hand, the implementation and easy accessibility to the CRISPR/Cas9 technology has allowed the generation of diverse molecular methodologies that constitute significant advances in the genome edition and its subsequent exploitation for agrarian and health purposes. Therefore, this technique is considered a revolutionary tool.

The major challenges for CRISPR/Cas9 technology will focus on two underlying aspects. First, the corresponding ethical or bioethical discussion, in order to demarcate what should or should not be done with this tool considering the risks that we could face by using promising technology, an even more when this is accessible and cheap. On the other hand, the legal consequences in terms of intellectual property that today literally generate wars between law firms and universities for the patents generated by thousands of investigations must be considered. Although many scientists consider CRISPR/Cas9 system as a "Holy Grail of genetic engineering," we must not lose sight of the objectivity and rationality when interpreting the consequences of its use. Additionally, demanding compliance with all the necessary safety steps before this technology becomes a trivial routine, especially if this tool is used for genome editing, and the genetic improvement of living beings must be imperative.

The features of the CRISPR/Cas9 system have allowed opening the possibility of using it to perform gene and cell therapy, in addition to its application in plant genetic improvement. In general, this technology has been used as a tool to perform point mutations, homologous recombination by HDR, and silencing and activation or repression of gene transcription. Thanks to these properties, its application has been possible for genetic monitoring, analysis of metabolic pathways, functional genomic research, generation of animal models, discovery of possible targets for disease treatments, and, even, correction of phenotypes. Another application of great importance that should continue to be developed is the generation of more precise and representative plant lines for the study of phytopathogenic diseases. Knockdown, knockout, and knocking models show the advantage of being able to be quickly and efficiently generated with this system. Also, CRISPR/Cas9 is considered a great biotechnological tool in the field of human therapies since its capacity to perform genetic level corrections/deletions, which is traduced in the possibility of regulating transcription or translation pathways.

In relation to the introduction of CRISPR/Cas9 in agricultural and environmental sciences, several studies recognize the possibilities of this technique to improve crop varieties [25, 80]. Uncertainty about safety and efficacy of genome editing requires evaluating its potential and utility by applying the precautionary principle. Research on this technology also unchains important legal and social debates among genetic engineering and genomic editing, in order to establish whether new mechanisms are needed to regulate research, confined use, voluntary release and if it is necessary to evaluate the possible impact on the environment just like in consumers' health, among other aspects. The application of the precautionary principle in any case must be done considering the available scientific evidence and raising the necessary social and economic considerations, in order to avoid a dogmatic interpretation that could undermine or stop scientific progress.

Nevertheless, despite the great potential of the CRISPR/Cas9 technique, it is also common to find evident limitations, since other alternatives have been proposed to improve genome editing with biotechnological processes [81]. Molecularly, the components of the CRISPR/Cas9 system are too large to be introduced into a viral genome (e.g.), and thus, they are most commonly used in gene therapy to transport foreign genetic material into human and plant cells. One solution for this problem is to use a smaller type of a Cas9 enzyme, obtained from *S. aureus* [82]. This enzyme is small enough to fit in the virus. The mini-Cas9 complex has been used in mice to correct the gene responsible for Duchenne muscular dystrophy [83].

The Cas9 enzyme not always cleavages where it is intended within the genome (a certain DNA sequence must be nearby for that to happen). This is easily accomplished in many genomes, but it may be a limitation in some experiments. Researchers are constantly looking for microbes to obtain enzymes with different genome characteristics to expand the number of sequences that can be modified. One of these enzymes is called Cpf1, and it can be an interesting alternative, since it is smaller than Cas9 and has different characteristics in its sequence that make it highly specific [84, 85]. Another enzyme called C2c2 is able to target RNA instead of DNA, which is why it has a great potential to study RNA and to fight plant viruses with this type of genomes [86].

Several laboratories apply CRISPR/Cas9 technology in order to eliminate specific regions in a gene sequence, thus repressing its function. Those who want to exchange a sequence for another face a more difficult task. When Cas9 cleavages the DNA, the cell makes mistakes by regrouping the loose ends, thus obtaining desired deletions. Researchers who want to rewrite a DNA sequence rely on different repair pathways that can insert new sequences (a process that occurs at a much lower frequency). Cas9 directs the sequence dictated by its guiding RNA, but does not cut it; instead, the bound enzyme changes the letters of DNA, ultimately producing a T where once there was a C [87].

In contrast to the above, recent new gene editing systems have been released using a protein called NgAgo to cleavage DNA at a predetermined site without the need for an RNA guide or a genome-specific neighbor sequence. Instead, the protein (of bacterial origin) is programmed using a short DNA sequence corresponding to the target sequence. However, laboratories have failed to reproduce the results so far, so the effectiveness of this technique cannot be affirmed [88]. There are also other genetic editing systems, some of which have existed for years. For example, scientists rely heavily on a system called lambda Red, which can be programmed to alter DNA sequences without the need for a RNA guide.

In light of the above considerations, we can finally conclude that the biotechnological tools that belong to cas9 toolbox that in synergism with new bioinformatic algorithms increase their potential in a specific and powerful way and help position this technology as a magnificent last generation method for genomic edition, which is considered a revolutionary scientific discovery for both basic and applied research including the field of plant biotechnology, even when there are inconclusive details of its application in the laboratory and very probably a gross ignorance of its nature, for now.

Acknowledgements

Thanks are to the General Directorate of Research (DGI) from Veracruz University and the General Directorate of Superior University Education (PRODEP). Our gratitude is also for Nestle Company through the Cacao Nestle Plan of Mexico. Finally, we are indebted to the reviewers for their useful and constructive comments and suggestions regarding this document.

Conflict of interest

The authors declare no conflict of interest regarding the conduct of this work and the results obtained from it.

Author details

Jorge Ricaño-Rodríguez[1]*, Jorge Suárez-Medellin[2], Eliezer Cocoletzi Vásquez[1], José M. Ramos-Prado[1] and Enrique Hipólito-Romero[1]

*Address all correspondence to: jricano@uv.mx

1 Center of EcoLiteracy and Dialogue of Knowledge, University of Veracruz, Xalapa, Veracruz, Mexico

2 Brain Research Center, University of Veracruz, Xalapa, Veracruz, Mexico

References

[1] Belhaj J, Chaparro-García A, Kamoun S, Patron NJ, Nekrasov V. Editing plant genomes with CRISPR/Cas9. Current Opinion in Biotechnology. 2015;**32**:76-84. DOI: 10.1016/j.copbio.2014.11.007

[2] Kunin V, Sorek R, Hugenholtz P. Evolutionary conservation of sequence and secondary structures in CRISPR repeats. Genome Biology. 2007;**8**:R61. DOI: 10.1186/gb-2007-8-4-r61

[3] Mojica FJ, Díez-Villaseñor C, García-Martínez J, Almendros C. Short motif sequences determine the targets of the prokaryotic CRISPR defense system. Microbiology. 2009;**155**: 733-740. DOI: 10.1099/mic.0.023960-0

[4] Wright AV, Nuñez JK, Doudna JA. Biology and applications of CRISPR systems: Harnessing nature's toolbox for genome engineering. Cell. 2016;**164**:29-44. DOI: 10.1016/j.cell.2015.12.035

[5] Makarova KS, Haft DH, Barrangou R, Brouns SJ, Charpentier E, Horvath P, et al. Evolution and classification of the CRISPR-Cas systems. Nature Reviews Microbiology. 2011;**9**: 467-477. DOI: 10.1038/nrmicro2577

[6] van der Oost J, Jore MM, Westra ER, Lundgren M, Brouns SJ. CRISPR-based adaptive and heritable immunity in prokaryotes. Trends in Biochemical Sciences. 2009;**34**:401-407

[7] Liu D, Hu R, Palla KJ, Tuskan GA, Yang X. Advances and perspectives on the use of CRISPR/Cas9 systems in plant genomics research. Current Opinion in Plant Biology. 2016; **30**:70-77. DOI: 10.1016/j.pbi.2016.01.007

[8] Liu X, Wu S, Xu J, Sui C, Wei J. Applications of CRISPR/Cas9 in plant biology. Acta Pharmaceutica Sinica B. 2017;**7**:292-302. DOI: 10.1016/j.apsb.2017.01.002

[9] Karvelis T, Gasiunas G, Young J, Bigelyte G, Silanskas A, Cigan M, et al. Rapid characterization of CRISPR-Cas9 protospacers adjacent motif sequence elements. Genome Biology. 2015;**16**:253. DOI: 10.1186/s13059-015-0818-7

[10] Ran FA, Cong L, Yan WX, Scott DA, Gootenberg JS, Kriz AJ, et al. In vivo genome editing using *Staphylococcus aureus* Cas9. Nature. 2015;**520**:186-191. DOI: 10.1038/nature14299

[11] Steinert J, Schiml S, Fauser F, Puchta H. Highly efficient heritable plant genome engineering using Cas9 orthologues from *Streptococcus thermophilus* and *Staphylococcus aureus*. The Plant Journal. 2015;**84**:1295-1305. DOI: 10.1111/tpj.13078

[12] Jacobs TB, Lafayette PR, Schmitz RJ, Parrott WA. Targeted genome modifications in soybean with CRISPR/Cas9. BMC Biotechnology. 2015;**15**:16. DOI: 10.1186/s12896-015-0131-2

[13] Lieber MR. The mechanism of double-strand DNA break repair by the nonhomologous DNA end joining pathway. Annual Review of Biochemistry. 2010;**79**:181-211. DOI: 10.1146/annurev.biochem.052308.093131

[14] Xie KB, Yang YN. RNA-guided genome editing in plants using a CRISPR-Cas system. Molecular Plant. 2013;**6**:1975-1983. DOI: 10.1093/mp/sst119

[15] Mojica F, Garcia-Martinez J, Soria E. Intervening sequences of regularly spaced prokaryotic repeats derive from foreign genetic elements. Journal of Molecular Evolution. 2005;**60**: 174-182. DOI: 10.1007/s00239-004-0046-3

[16] Lindhout BI, Fransz P, Tessadori F, Meckel T, Hooykaas PJ, van der Zaal BJ. Live cell imaging of repetitive DNA sequences via GFP-tagged polydactyl zinc finger proteins. Nucleic Acids Research. 2007;**35**:e107. DOI: 10.1093/nar/gkm618

[17] Miyanari Y, Ziegler-Birling C, Torres-Padilla ME. Live visualization of chromatin dynamics with fluorescent TALEs. Nature Structural & Molecular Biology. 2013;**20**:1321-1324. DOI: 10.1038/nsmb.2680

[18] Jinek M, Jiang F, Taylor DW, Sternberg SH, Kaya E, Ma E, et al. Structures of Cas9 endonucleases reveal RNA-mediated conformational activation. Science. 2014;**343**(6176): 1247997. DOI: 10.1126/science.1247997

[19] Jiang F, Doudna JA. CRISPR-Cas9 structures and mechanisms. Annual Review of Biophysics. 2017;**46**:505-529. DOI: 10.1146/annurev-biophys-062215-010822

[20] Nishimasu H, Ran FA, Hsu PD, Konermann S, Shehata SI, Dohmae N, et al. Crystal structure of Cas9 in complex with guide RNA and target DNA. Cell. 2014;**156**:935-949. DOI: 10.1016/j.cell.2014.02.001

[21] Song G, Jia M, Chen K, Kong X, Khattak B, Xie C, et al. CRISPR/Cas9: A powerful tool for crop genome editing. The Crop Journal. 2016;**4**:75-82. DOI: 10.1016/j.cj.2015.12.002

[22] Puchta H. The repair of double stranded DNA breaks in plants: Mechanisms and consequences for genome evolution. Journal of Experimental Botany. 2005;**56**:1-14. DOI: 10.1093/jxb/eri025

[23] Gilbert LA, Horlbeck MA, Adamson B, Villalta JE, Chen YW, Whitehead EH, et al. Genome-scale CRISPR-mediated control of gene expression and activation. Cell. 2014;**159**:1-15. DOI: 10.1016/j.cell.2014.09.029

[24] Rusk N. CRISPRs and epigenome editing. Nature Methods. 2014;**11**:28. DOI: 10.1038/nmeth.2775

[25] Paul JW 3rd, Qi Y. CRISPR/Cas9 for plant genome editing: Accomplishments, problems and prospects. Plant Cell Reports. 2016;**35**:1417-1427. DOI: 10.1007/s00299-016-1985-z

[26] Fu Y, Foden JA, Khayter C, Maeder ML, Reyon D, Joung JK, et al. High-frequency off-target mutagenesis induced by CRISPR-Cas nucleases in human cells. Nature Biotechnology. 2013;**31**:822-826. DOI: 10.1038/nbt.2623

[27] Mali P, Aach J, Stranges PB, Esvelt KM, Moosburner M, Kosuri S, et al. CAS9 transcriptional activators for target specificity screening and paired nickases for cooperative genome engineering. Nature Biotechnology. 2013;**31**:833-838. DOI: 10.1038/nbt.2675

[28] Bortesi L, Fischer R. The CRISPR/Cas9 system for plant genome editing and beyond. Biotechnology Advances. 2015;**33**:41-52. DOI: 10.1016/jbiotechadv.2014.12.006

[29] Sander JD, Dahlborg EJ, Goodwin MJ, Cade L, Zhang F, Cifuentes D, et al. Selection-free zinc-finger-nuclease engineering by context-dependent assembly (CoDA). Nature Methods. 2011;**8**:67-69. DOI: 10.1038/nmeth.1542

[30] Ramirez CL, Foley JE, Wright DA, Müller-Lerch F, Rahman SH, Cornu TI, et al. Unexpected failure rates for modular assembly of engineered zinc fingers. Nature Methods. 2008;**5**:374-375. DOI: 10.1038/nmeth0508-374

[31] Doyle EL, Booher NJ, Standage DS, Voytas DF, Brendel VP, Vandyk JK, et al. TAL Effector-Nucleotide Targeter (TALEN-NT) 2.0: Tools for TAL effector design and target prediction. Nucleic Acids Research. 2012;**40**:117-122. DOI: 10.1093/nar/gks608

[32] Gupta RM, Musunuru K. Expanding the genetic editing tool kit: ZFNs, TALENs, and CRISPR-Cas9. Journal of Clinical Investigation. 2014;**124**(10):4154-4161. DOI: 10.1172/JCI72992

[33] Reyon D, Tsai SQ, Khayter C, Foden JA, Sander JD, Joung JK. FLASH assembly of TALENs for high-throughput genome editing. Nature Biotechnology. 2012;**30**:460-465. DOI: 10.1038/nbt.2170

[34] Holkers M, Maggio I, Liu J, Janssen JM, Miselli F, Mussolino C, et al. Differential integrity of TALE nuclease genes following adenoviral and lentiviral vector gene transfer into human cells. Nucleic Acids Research. 2013;**41**:e63. DOI: 10.1093/nar/gks1446

[35] Yang L, Guell M, Byrne S, Yang JL, De Los Angeles A, Mali P, et al. Optimization of scarless human stem cell genome editing. Nucleic Acids Research. 2013;**41**:9049-9061. DOI: 10.1093/nar/gkt555

[36] Li J-F, Aach J, Norville JE, McCormack M, Zhang D, Bush J, et al. Multiplex and homologous recombination-mediated genome editing in *Arabidopsis* and *Nicotiana benthamiana* using guide RNA and Cas9. Nature Biotechnology. 2013;**31**:688-691. DOI: 10.1038/nbt.2654

[37] Jiang W, Bikard D, Cox D, Zhang F, Marraffini LA. RNA-guided editing of bacterial genomes using CRISPR-Cas systems. Nature Biotechnology. 2013a;**31**:233-239. DOI: 10.1038/nbt.2508

[38] Jiang W, Zhou H, Bi H, Fromm M, Yang B, Weeks DP. Demonstration of CRISPR/Cas9/sgRNA-mediated targeted gene modification in *Arabidopsis*, tobacco, sorghum and rice. Nucleic Acids Research. 2013;**41**:e188. DOI: 10.1093/nar/gkt780

[39] Upadhyay SK, Kumar J, Alok A, Tuli R. RNA-guided genome editing for target gene mutations in wheat. G3: Genes, Genomes, Genetics. 2013;**3**:2233-2238. DOI: 10.1534/g3.113.008847

[40] Shan Q, Wang Y, Li J, Zhang Y, Chen K, Liang Z, et al. Targeted genome modification of crop plants using a CRISPR-Cas system. Nature Biotechnology. 2013;**31**:686-688. DOI: 10.1038/nbt.2650

[41] Liang Z, Zhang K, Chen K, Gao C. Targeted mutagenesis in *Zea mays* using TALENs and the CRISPR/Cas system. Journal of Genetics and Genomics. 2014;**41**:63-68. DOI: 10.1016/j.jgg.2013.12.001

[42] Jia H, Wang N. Targeted genome editing of sweet orange using Cas9/sgRNA. PLoS One. 2014;**9**:e93806. DOI: 10.1371/journal.pone.0093806

[43] Huang S, Weigel D, Beachy RN, Li J. A proposed regulatory framework for genome-edited crops. Nature Genetics. 2016;**48**(2):109-111. DOI: 10.1038/ng.3484

[44] Nekrasov V, Staskawicz B, Weigel D, Jones JDG, Kamoun S. Targeted mutagenesis in the model plant *Nicotiana benthamiana* using Cas9 RNA-guided endonuclease. Nature Biotechnology. 2013;**31**(8):691-693. DOI: 10.1038/nbt.2655

[45] Zhou H, Liu B, Weeks DP, Spalding MH, Yang B. Large chromosomal deletions and heritable small genetic changes induced by CRISPR/Cas9 in rice. Nucleic Acids Research. 2014;**42**(17):10903-10914. DOI: 10.1093/nar/gku806

[46] Endo M, Mikami M, Toki S. Multigene Knockout Utilizing Off-Target Mutations of the CRISPR/Cas9 System in Rice. Plant and Cell Physiology. 2015;**56**(1):41-47. DOI: 10.1093/pcp/pcu154

[47] Xu RF, Li H, Qin RY, Li J, Qiu CH, Yang YC, et al. Generation of inheritable and "transgene clean" targeted genome-modified rice in later generations using the CRISPR/Cas9 system. Scientific Reports. 2015;**5**:11491. DOI: 10.1038/srep11491

[48] Lu Y, Zhu JK. Precise editing of a target base in the rice genome using a modified CRISPR/Cas9 system. Molecular Plant. 2017;**10**:523-525. DOI: 10.1016/j.molp.2016.11.013

[49] Li J, Meng X, Zong Y, Chen K, Zhang H, Liu J, et al. Gene replacements and insertions in rice by intron targeting using CRISPR-Cas9. Nature Plants. 2016;**2**:16139. DOI: 10.1038/NPLANTS.2016.139

[50] Sun Y, Zhang X, Wu C, He Y, Ma Y, Guo X, et al. Engineering herbicide-resistant rice plants through CRISPR/Cas9-mediated homologous recombination of acetolactate synthase. Molecular Plant. 2016;**9**:628-631. DOI: 10.1016/j.molp.2016.01.00

[51] Shimatani Z, Kashojiya S, Takayama M, Terada R, Arazoe T, Ishii H, et al. Targeted base editing in rice and tomato using a CRISPR-Cas9 cytidine deaminase fusion. Nature Biotechnology. 2017;**35**:441-443. DOI: 10.1038/nbt.3833

[52] Wang F, Wang C, Liu P, Lei C, Hao W, Gao Y, et al. Enhanced rice blast resistance by CRISPR/Cas9-targeted mutagenesis of the erf transcription factor gene OsERF922. PLoS One. 2016;**11**(4):e0154027. DOI: 10.1371/journal.pone.0154027

[53] Gil-Humanes J, Wang Y, Liang Z, Shan Q, Ozuna CV, Sánchez-León S, et al. High-efficiency gene targeting in hexaploid wheat using DNA replicons and CRISPR/Cas9. The Plant Journal. 2017;**89**:1251-1262. DOI: 10.1111/tpj.13446

[54] Zhang Y, Liang Z, Zong Y, Wang Y, Liu J, Chen K, et al. Efficient and transgene-free genome editing in wheat through transient expression of CRISPR/Cas9 DNA or RNA. Nature Communications. 2016;**7**:12617. DOI: 10.1038/ncomms12617

[55] Liang Z, Chen K, Li T, Zhang Y, Wang Y, Zhao Q, et al. Efficient DNA-free genome editing of bread wheat using CRISPR/Cas9 ribonucleoprotein complexes. Nature Communications. 2016;**8**:14261. DOI: 10.1038/ncomms14261

[56] Wang Y, Cheng X, Shan Q, Zhang Y, Liu J, Gao C, et al. Simultaneous editing of three homoeoalleles in hexaploid bread wheat confers heritable resistance to powdery mildew. Nature Biotechnology. 2014;**32**:947-951. DOI: 10.1038/nbt.2969

[57] Sun X, Hu Z, Chen R, Jiang Q, Song G, Zhang H, et al. Targeted mutagenesis in soybean using the CRISPR-Cas9 system. Scientific Reports. 2015;**5**:10342. DOI: 10.1038/srep10342

[58] Cai Y, Chen L, Liu X, Sun S, Wu C, Jiang B, et al. CRISPR/Cas9-mediated genome editing in soybean hairy roots. PLoS One. 2015;**10**(8):e0136064. DOI: 10.1371/journal.pone.0136064

[59] Char SN, Neelakandan AK, Nahampun H, Frame B, Main M, Spalding MH, et al. An Agrobacterium-delivered CRISPR/Cas9 system for high-frequency targeted mutagenesis in maize. Plant Biotechnology Journal. 2017;**15**:257-268. DOI: 10.1111/pbi.12611

[60] Svitashev S, Schwartz C, Lenderts B, Young JK, Cigan M. Genome editing in maize directed by CRISPR–Cas9 ribonucleoprotein complexes. Nature Communications. 2016; **7**:13274. DOI: 10.1038/ncomms13274

[61] Shi J, Gao H, Wang H, Lafitte HR, Archibald RL, Yang M, et al. ARGOS8 variants generated by CRISPR-Cas9 improve maize grain yield under field drought stress conditions. Plant Biotechnology Journal. 2017;**15**:207-216. DOI: 10.1111/pbi.12603

[62] Brooks C, Nekrasov V, Lippman ZB, Eck JV. Efficient gene editing in tomato in the first generation using the clustered regularly interspaced short palindromic repeats/CRISPR-associated9 System. Plant Physiology. 2014;**166**:1292-1297. DOI: 10.1104/pp.114.247577

[63] Pan C, Ye L, Qin L, Liu X, He Y, Wang J, et al. CRISPR/Cas9-mediated efficient and heritable targeted mutagenesis in tomato plants in the first and later generations. Scientific Reports. 2016;**6**:24765. DOI: 10.1038/srep24765

[64] Ito Y, Nishizawa-Yokoi A, Endo M, Mikami M, Toki S. CRISPR/Cas9-mediated mutagenesis of the *RIN* locus that regulates tomato fruit ripening. Biochemical and Biophysical Research Communications. 2015;**467**(1):76-82. DOI: 10.1016/j.bbrc.2015.09.117

[65] Ueta R, Abe C, Watanabe T, Sugano SS, Ishihara R, Ezura H, et al. Rapid breeding of parthenocarpic tomato plants using CRISPR/Cas9. Scientific Reports. 2017;**7**:507. DOI: 10.1038/s41598-017-00501-4

[66] Gao J, Wang G, Ma S, Xie X, Wu X, Zhang X, et al. CRISPR/Cas9-mediated targeted mutagenesis in *Nicotiana tabacum*. Plant Molecular Biology. 2015;**87**:99-110. DOI: 10.1007/s11103-014-0263-0

[67] Wang S, Zhang S, Wang W, Xiong X, Meng F, Cui X. Efficient targeted mutagenesis in potato by the CRISPR/Cas9 system. Plant Cell Reports. 2015;**34**(9):1473-1476. DOI: 10.1007/s00299-015-1816-7

[68] Zhang B, Yang X, Yang C, Li M, Guo Y. Exploiting the CRISPR/Cas9 system for targeted genome mutagenesis in petunia. Scientific Reports. 2016;**6**:20315. DOI: 10.1038/srep20315

[69] Ali Z, Abulfaraj A, Idris A, Ali S, Tashkandi M, Mahfouz MM. CRISPR/Cas9-mediated viral interference in plants. Genome Biology. 2015;**16**:238. DOI: 10.1186/s13059-015-0799-6

[70] Pyott DE, Sheehan E, Molnar A. Engineering of CRISPR/Cas9-mediated potyvirus resistance in transgene-free Arabidopsis plants. Molecular Plant Pathology. 2016;**17**(8):1276-1288. DOI: 10.1111/mpp.12417

[71] Osakabe Y, Watanabe T, Sugano SS, Ueta R, Ishihara R Shinozaki K, Osakabe K. Optimization of CRISPR/Cas9 genome editing to modify abiotic stress responses in plants. Scientific Reports. 2016;**6**:26685. DOI: 10.1038/srep26685

[72] Jiang WZ, Henry IM, Lynagh PG, Comai L, Cahoon EB, Weeks DP. Significant enhancement of fatty acid composition in seeds of the allohexaploid, *Camelina sativa*, using CRISPR/Cas9 gene editing. Plant Biotechnology Journal. 2017;**15**:648-657. DOI: 10.1111/pbi.12663

[73] Morineau C, Bellec Y, Tellier F, Gissot L, Kelemen Z, Nogué F, et al. Selective gene dosage by CRISPR-Cas9 genome editing in hexaploid *Camelina sativa*. Plant Biotechnology Journal. 2017;**15**:729-739. DOI: 10.1111/pbi.12671

[74] Chandrasekaran J, Brumin M, Wolf D, Leibman D, Klap C, Pearlsman M, et al. Development of broad virus resistance in non-transgenic cucumber using CRISPR/Cas9 technology. Molecular Plant Pathology. 2016;**17**(7):1140-1153. DOI: 10. 1111/mpp.12375

[75] Malnoy M, Viola R, Jung MH, Koo OJ, Kim S, Kim JS, et al. DNA-free genetically edited grapevine and apple protoplast using CRISPR/Cas9 ribonucleoproteins. Frontiers in Plant Science. 2016;**7**:1904. DOI: 10.3389/fpls.2016.01904

[76] Lawrenson T, Shorinola O, Stacey N, Li C, Østergaard L, Patron N, et al. Induction of targeted, heritable mutations in barley and *Brassica oleracea* using RNA-guided Cas9 nuclease. Genome Biology. 2015;**16**:258. DOI: 10.1186/s13059-015-0826-7

[77] Tian S, Jiang L, Gao Q, Zhang J, Zong M, Zhang H, et al. Efficient CRISPR/Cas9-based gene knockout in watermelon. Plant Cell Reports. 2017;**36**(3):399-406. DOI: 10.1007/s00299-016-2089-5

[78] Fan D, Liu T, Li C, Jiao B, Li S, Hou Y, et al. Efficient CRISPR/Cas9-mediated targeted mutagenesis in *populus* in the first generation. Scientific Reports. 2015;**5**:12217. DOI: 10.1038/srep1221

[79] Wolt JD, Wang K, Yang B. The regulatory status of genome-edited crops. Plant Biotechnology Journal. 2016;**14**:510-518. DOI: 10.1111/pbi.12444

[80] Khatodia S, Bhatotia K, Passricha N, Khurana SM, Tuteja N. The CRISPR /Cas genome-editing tool: Application in improvement of crops. Frontiers in Plant Science. 2016;**7**:1-13. DOI: 10.3389/fpls.2016.00506

[81] Ledford H. Beyond CRISPR: A guide to the many other ways to edit a genome. Nature. 2016;**11, 536**:136-137. DOI: 10.1038/536136b

[82] Marraffini LA, Sontheimer EJ. CRISPR interference limits horizontal gene transfer in Staphylococci by targeting DNA. Science. 2008;**322**:1843-1845. DOI: 10.1126/Science.1165771

[83] Nelson CE, Hakim CH, Ousterout DG, Thakore PI, Moreb EA, Castellanos Rivera RM, et al. In vivo genome editing improves muscle function in a mouse model of Duchenne muscular dystrophy. Science. 2016;**22**(351):403-407. DOI: 10.1126/science.aad5143

[84] Kim D, Kim J, Hur JK, Been KW, Yoon SH, Kim JS. Genome-wide analysis reveals specificities of Cpf1 endonucleases in human cells. Nature Biotechnology. 2016;**9**(34):888. DOI: 10.1038/nbt0816-888a

[85] Kleinstiver BP, Tsai SQ, Prew MS, Nguyen N, Welch MM, Lopez JM, et al. Genome-wide specificities of CRISPR-Cas Cpf1 nucleases in human cells. Nature Biotechnology. 2016; **34**(8):869-874. DOI: 10.1038/nbt.3620

[86] Abudayyeh OO, Gootenberg JS, Konermann S, Joung J, Slaymaker IM, Cox DB, et al. C2c2 is a single-component programmable RNA-guided RNA-targeting CRISPR effector. Science. 2016;**5**(353):aaf5573. DOI: 10.1126/science.aaf5573

[87] Komor AC, Kim YB, Packer MS, Zuris JA, Liu DR. Programmable editing of a target base in genomic DNA without double-stranded DNA cleavage. Nature. 2016;**533**(7603):420-424. DOI: 10.1038/nature17946

[88] Gao F, Shen XZ, Jiang F, Wu Y, Han C. DNA-guided genome editing using the *Natronobacterium gregoryi* Argonaute. Nature Biotechnology. 2016;**34**:768-773. DOI: 10.1038/nbt.3547

Chapter 4

Technical Advances in Chloroplast Biotechnology

Muhammad Sarwar Khan, Ghulam Mustafa and
Faiz Ahmad Joyia

Additional information is available at the end of the chapter

http://dx.doi.org/10.5772/intechopen.81240

Abstract

Chloroplasts are highly organized cellular organelles after master organelle nucleus. They not only play a central role in photosynthesis but are also involved in several crucial cellular activities. Advancements in molecular biology and transgenic technology have further groomed importance of the organelle, and they are the most ideal ones for the expression of transgene. No doubt, limitations are there, but still research is advancing to resolve those. Certain valuable traits have been engineered for improved agronomic performance of crop plants. Industrial enzymes and therapeutic proteins have been expressed using plastid transformation system. Synthetic biology has been explored to play a key role in engineering metabolic pathways. Further, producing dsRNA in a plant's chloroplast rather than in its cellular cytoplasm is more effective way to address desired traits. In this chapter, we highlight technological advancements in chloroplast biotechnology and its implication to develop biosafe engineered plants.

Keywords: chloroplast biotechnology, value-added crops, RNAi, trouble-rescue organelles, plastid functional genomics

1. Introduction

Food security is a long-lasting challenge for the growing world and is becoming more alarming in the developing countries where one out of every nine people is malnourished. So-called processing (polishing, milling, and pearling) of the cereals makes them even poorer in micronutrients [1]. Climate change is another challenge that poses continuous stress on the crop productivity. Sharply decreasing arable soils and use of heavy inputs to get high crop yield are further deteriorating our environment and quality of available food. All this demands availability of improved crop cultivars having ability to perform in the changing climate scenario and even with balanced dose of micronutrients. Gene revolution is the only hope for second green revolution to attain these ideal crop cultivars [2]. Since the commercialization of transgenic crops in 1994, the area under GM crops is sharply increasing and has now increased to 180 million hectares. This includes crops for improved agronomic traits (herbicide tolerance and insect resistance, salinity and drought tolerance, and efficient nutrient utilization), enhanced level of micronutrients, and for the expression of therapeutic proteins and industrially important enzymes. At the same time, emotional or obsolete arguments are there to oppose the use of GM (genetically modified) products. Opponents of GM crops have straightforwardly rejected genetically modified products and have produced questionable scientific data to ban their commercialization. Plastid biotechnology has emerged as a competent field of research having potential to address all of the questions raised by the opponents of GM crops [3]. This chapter highlights significance of plastid transgenic technology to develop valuable crop plants. Further, technological advancements have been discussed to get an update about the recent research to resolve existing bottlenecks in the development and commercialization of transplastomic plants.

2. Chloroplast biotechnology—an overview

Transgenic technology is the technology of the day to develop crop plants with desired traits but crucial traits need to be engineered through plastid genome instead of nuclear genome [4]. It is an amazing organelle where more than 120 genes from various sources have been integrated and expressed. This organellar genome has well been explored for a wide variety of applications including crops with elevated level of resistance against biotic (insects, bacterial, viral, and fungal diseases) and abiotic stresses (salinity, drought, and cold); phytoremediation of toxic metals, cytoplasmic male sterility [5]; and production of biopharmaceuticals, vaccine antigens, industrial enzymes, biomaterials, and biofuel [6]. Hyperexpression of recombinant protein in plant expression system is only possible through plastid transformation. The high ploidy number of the plastid genome results in higher level of protein expression, and up to 70% total soluble protein is reported to be produced in tobacco [7]. Moreover, hyperexpression of therapeutic proteins and vaccine antigens in chloroplasts (leaves), leucoplasts (roots), or chromoplasts (fruits) makes it ideal organelle for the oral delivery of vaccine antigens against tetanus, cholera, anthrax, canine parvovirus, and plague [8]. Other salient advantages include possibility of multigene engineering, absence of gene silencing, position effect, epigenetic, complete absence of pleiotropic effects due to subcellular compartmentalization, and transgene containment due to maternal inheritance of plastids in most of the crops [9].

Plastid transformation was first established in unicellular green algae (*Chlamydomonas reinhardtii*) followed by model tobacco plant. It has now been well established in economically valuable crops (rice, brassica, cotton, carrot, spinach, lettuce, etc.) and even in woody plant like popular. Small circular plastid genome (plastome) facilitates targeted engineering, which has been exploited not only for basic research but also for the applied research [10]. Most of the genes present in plastome have been characterized through functional genomics. Organellar transcription and translation have been thoroughly elucidated to understand transcriptional and translational machinery of the plastids. Even the proteins involved in cross-talk between chloroplast and nucleus have been worked out. Further, plastid transformation is the most ideal technology to develop marker-free transgenic plants where antibiotic resistance genes, used for the selection of putative transformants, are not acceptable by the ultimate consumer. Different techniques have been developed to produce marker-free plants in order to facilitate the acceptance of transplastomic crops. In spite of so many advantages of plastid transformation technology, there are still difficulties impeding expansion of this technology to economically valuable crops particularly monocots. These include lack of species-specific regulatory sequences, inefficient selection system, metabolic burden in case of hyperexpression and unavailability of green plastids in monocots.

3. Making better crops through chloroplast engineering

It is predicted that sharply increasing population necessitates an increase in crop yield at 30% per annum. In this scenario, chloroplast biotechnology is the most ideal approach to develop crop plants with improved photosynthetic performance, enhanced nutritional value, improved agronomic traits, and producing valuable fatty acids. Plastid transformation was first established in flowering plants almost 30 years ago. Though it has been extended to other crop plants, most of the studies have been conducted in tobacco, which is nonfood nonfeed crop. This demands further efforts by the scientific community to engineer plastid genome of valuable crop plants for desired traits, leading to increased quality and quantity of food.

Most of the efforts to increase crop productivity had been made to improve photosynthetic performance of the plants. RuBisCO (the core enzyme of photosynthesis), large subunit, is encoded by chloroplasts, whereas small subunit is encoded by nuclease, which is then imported to chloroplast. Efforts have been made to engineer RuBisCO large subunit, small subunit, or both. Lin [11] attempted to express complete RuBisCO protein in tobacco from *Synechococcus elongatus* by disrupting the host native enzyme. CO2 fixation rate and carboxylase activity of the RuBisCO were increased, especially at higher concentrations of CO_2. Hence, photosynthetic performance can be improved by introducing more competent complete photosynthetic system into a plant. Raising concentration of CO_2 in plastids is another possibility strategy, to improve photosynthetic carbon fixation and crop productivity. Cyanobacterial bicarbonate transporter was expressed in tobacco plastid genome, but any considerable improvement in photosynthetic performance was not observed. Expression of fructose-1,6-sedoheptulose-1,7-bisphosphatase in lettuce and tobacco chloroplasts appeared to increase productivity of engineered plants. Likewise, chloroplast-encoded chlB gene from *Pinus thunbergii* was found to promote root growth and early chlorophyll pigment development in tobacco [12]. Hence, research is in progress to engineer C3 plants to C4 by manipulating RuBisCO large subunit and photorespiratory pathway for enhanced biomass production [13].

Insect resistant crops had successfully been grown in the field since 1994. Resistance development against Bt crops is an emerging concern, which needs to be addressed through high-dose strategy and gene pyramiding. Another possibility to develop insect-resistant transplastomic plants is the upregulation of their pathogen defense mechanisms. Expression of β-glucosidase in tobacco plastome showed not only growth of the plants but also more resistance against insect pests [14]. A novel non-Bt-type insect resistance strategy has been evaluated by expressing dsRNA, targeting an essential insect gene in transplastomic plants. Disruption of target gene by RNA interference resulted in 100% mortality in adult beetles and in the larvae within 5 days of feeding [15]. Expression of agglutinin gene (pta) in leaf chloroplasts resulted in broad spectrum resistance against lepidopteran insects, aphids, and viral and bacterial pathogens [16]. A gene stack comprising CeCPI (sporamin, taro cystatin) gene from sweet potato and chitinase from *Paecilomyces javanicus* was introduced into tobacco, and resultant plants showed resistance not only against various pests and diseases but also against salinity, osmotic stress, and oxidative stress [17]. Expression of osmoprotectant (yeast trehalose phosphate synthase) in tobacco plastids resulted in 20-fold higher trehalose accumulation; as a result, plants were tolerant to drought and osmotic stress [18]. The overexpression of *mdar* transgene in tobacco plastids and the fusion of such chloroplasts to Petunia cells were suggested to possibly protect the plants against oxidative stress. Oxidative stress tolerance was also enhanced in transplastomic tobacco plants expressing flavodoxin (fld) from cyanobacteria. Transplastomic plants overexpressing panD not only appeared to produce 30–40% higher biomass but also appeared to be more tolerant to increased heat stress. Similarly, expression of arabitol dehydrogenase (*ArDH)* in tobacco chloroplasts enabled them to survive even at 400 mM NaCl [19]. Chilling tolerance as well as growth was observed to be increased in tropical forage *Stylosanthes guianensis* expressing chloroplast protein 12 [20]. Recently, plastid transformation has been reported in a valuable vegetable *Momordica charantia* [21], marine microalga *Nannochloropsis oceanica* [22], and *Cyanidioschyzon merolae* [23], a red alga having ability to survive in high sulfur acidic hot spring environments. This may open new horizons in understanding stress adaptability and role of transplastomic technology in developing stress-tolerant plants.

4. Chloroplasts as trouble-rescue organelles

Chloroplasts not only are the central hubs for photosynthesis but also have evolved as fundamental trouble-rescue organelles. Recent studies have revealed that chloroplasts play a key role in switching plants from vegetative mode to defense mode. In addition to intraorganellar functions, they also play crucial role in the regulation of extraorganellar processes such as plant stress response, apoptosis, and immunity. Both of the cellular organelles (chloroplast and mitochondria) evoke their own particular Ca^{2+} signals [24], have their own Ca^{2+} binding proteins, and Ca^{2+} sensors, which are expected to play a significant role in Ca^{2+} signaling within the plant cell [25]. As a result, they have capacity to sequester and serve as sink for Ca^{2+}, which plays a key role in physiological and environmental responses of eukaryotic cells.

Chloroplasts are important intracellular calcium (Ca^{2+}) stores and may accumulate up to 15 mM or even higher. Most of the plastidic Ca^{2+} resides within the stroma or thylakoid membranes through interaction with calcium-binding proteins [26]. The concentration of free calcium was found to be very low when determined by targeting apoaequorin to the stroma of tobacco chloroplasts [27]. Hence, stroma is not the major sequester of Ca^{2+} in chloroplasts. This helped to elucidate that chloroplasts have their own active transporters on the envelope membranes, which help them to accumulate high concentrations of Ca^{2+} within the thylakoid membranes or some other unidentified Ca^{2+} stores. Identification of CAS (high capacity Ca^{2+}-binding protein) in the thylakoid membranes of *Arabidopsis thaliana* revealed out that active calcium uptake machinery is present on the membranes; so, the thylakoid membrane may be the major sequester of Ca^{2+} in chloroplasts [28]. It was further elucidated that activity of these transporters is regulated by light or photosynthesis, so chloroplasts take up calcium during the day and store it in the lumen or some identified sequestering sites. During the night, Ca^{2+} is released from the store houses for long-lasting, dark-induced Ca^{2+} signals; hence, sensing of photoperiod and light/dark transition seems to be regulated by Ca^{2+} signaling. In addition to light, Ca^{2+} signaling is also influenced by other abiotic stimuli (salinity, cold) and hence plays some crucial role in stress tolerance as well.

An active Ca^{2+} uptake machinery is present in chloroplast, which is regulated by transporters. Much research has not been conducted on these transporters; as a result, only few are known, whereas others are still to be elucidated. Two potential membrane transporters (Ca^{2+}-ATPase) in *Arabidopsis* are AtACA1 and AtHMA1. AtACA1 is an autoinhibited Ca^{2+} transporter, which is predicted to be targeted to the chloroplasts. It is specifically expressed in the root and is then localized to endoplasmic reticulum or tonoplast. AtHMA1 is a heavy metal P-type ATPase in the chloroplast envelope and plays an important role in calcium transportation [29]. Recently, another transporter AtGLR3.4 (glutamate receptor) has been explored to form Ca^{2+} permeable nonselective cation channels and is localized in the chloroplasts [30]. In addition, two MscS homologs, localized in the chloroplast, have also been evaluated to be essential for plastidic osmoregulation [31]. Since these transporters play a key role in the sequestration of calcium ions into the thylakoid lumen, Ca^{2+}/H^{+} antiporter also plays a significant role in Ca^{2+} uptake via thylakoid proton gradient. Pea thylakoid protein (PPF1) is another candidate calcium transporter at thylakoid membrane, which has been found to enhance Ca^{2+} currents when tested in human cultured cells. These findings demonstrate that Ca^{2+}-binding protein and Ca^{2+} transporters play a significant role in immune signal transduction pathway. Anyhow, most of the genes involved in these pathways are still to be elucidated.

5. Advances in plastid functional genomics

Plastids are known to get evolved from primitive cyanobacteria through a process known as endosymbiosis [32]. Although plastid genomes are much smaller as compared to their cyanobacterial progenitors, similarities in gene sequence as well as genome topology are evident. Just like cyanobacterial genome, plastid genomes are tightly packed with genes as a circular molecule [33]. *In vivo* genes of plastid may be present as a linear molecule or a complex branched form, and many copies of plastid genome can be harbor in each organelle. Size of plastid genomes varies from <100 to >1000 kbp (kilobase pair). The region of small single copy (SSC) and large single copy (LSC) are separated by two inverted repeats (IRs) present in the plastid genome (**Figure 1**). The thymine and adenine residues are often rich in plastid genome; a reductive evolution is also seen in those of mitochondrial genomes and bacterial endosymbionts [34]. Noncoding DNAs are abundantly present in some plastid genomes, while the others have self-splicing introns. The genome of some dinoflagellates spreads across a sea of minicircles; recently, multiple linear chromosomes formed a hairpin structure, which have been found in the plastid genome of certain green algae [35].

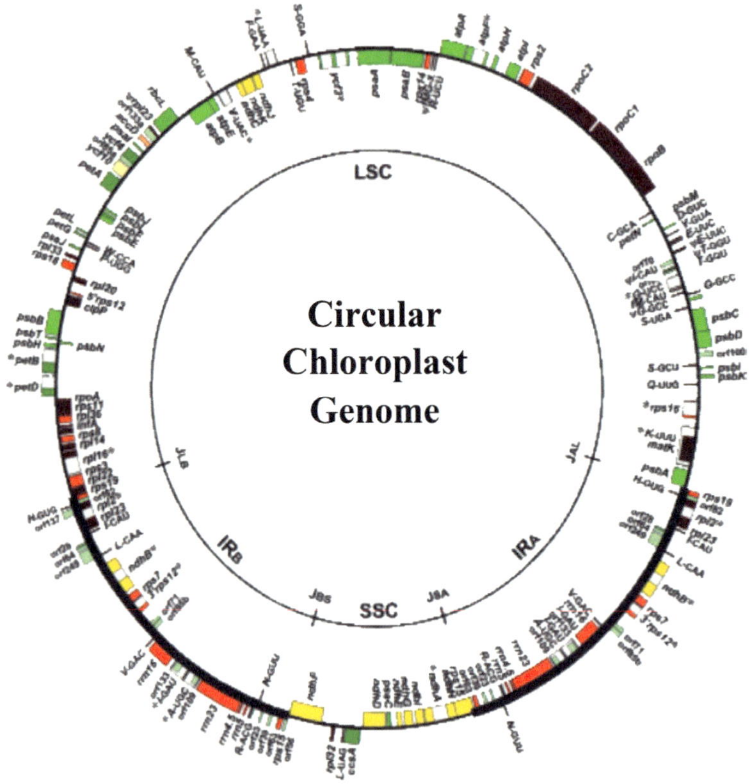

Figure 1. Circular map of chloroplast genome showing one large single copy (LSC), one small single copy (SSC), and two inverted repeats (IRa and IRb).

A huge portion of the cyanobacterium derivative genes required for plastid function now exist in the nucleus, having transferred through a process known as endosymbiotic gene transfer (EGT). Subsequently, most of the plastome proteins are introduced posttranslationally. Nevertheless, genomes of plastid normally encode some of their own processing machinery, including ribosomal proteins, ribosomal RNAs, bacterial RNAs polymerase, and tRNAs—however, land plants also have nuclear-encoded plastid RNA polymerases. Remarkably, genome of plastid also encodes many photosynthesis components, such as proteins of photosystem I and II (e.g., *psbA* gene of photosystem II coding for the D1 unit) as well as cytochrome *b6f*, which facilitates electron transfer between both photosystems I and II [36].

6. Role of synthetic biology in engineering plastid metabolic pathways

Though it is the beginning of plastid synthetic biology, advancements are being made to develop the essential tools regarding transgene expression control in chloroplast genome [37]. Currently, most recombinant expression in the plastids involves single-gene constructs created using conventional restriction enzyme-based cloning approaches. This limits the rate at which new transplastomic lines can be produced and tested, and in particular, how many different permutations of constructs (different promoters, coding variants, regulatory elements, etc.) can be evaluated. Currently, various synthetic biology principles are being applied to plastome engineering with the adoption of assembly standards such as Golden Gate and the creation of libraries of validated DNA parts that allow rapid one-step assembly of all the parts [38–40]. More ambitious design strategies involving extensive redesign of the plastome *in silico* are expected to be optimized and validated. Some of the foreseen strategies include removal of large tracts of nonessential DNA [41], refactoration of numerous essential endogenous genes into functional clusters [42], and synchronized engineering of multiple transgenes into different loci. The assembly and delivery of such synthetic genomes is technically feasible, as shown by O'Neill et al. [37], who demonstrated that the entire *C. reinhardtii* plastome could be assembled in yeast and transformed into *C. reinhardtii* by microparticle bombardment. Plastidic intercistronic expression elements (IEEs) can be used for the expression of synthetic operons [43]. The challenge is to develop selection strategies that allow the clean replacement of the endogenous plastome with the synthetic version without undesirable recombination events between the two, resulting in the creation of chimeric plastomes.

Another challenge is to improve the product yield significantly through the use of synthetic cis elements to drive expression. Currently, the promoter and 5′ UTR used to express transgenes are derived from endogenous photosynthetic genes. In some cases, expression levels can be improved by using the stronger promoter from the gene for the 16S ribosomal RNA fused to the 5′ UTR of a photosynthetic gene [44]. However, more often it is the performance of the 5′ UTR that is the bottleneck [45], with the efficiency of translation constrained by either the same feedback regulation that prevents the overaccumulation of individual photosynthetic subunits in the absence of their assembly partners (so-called "control by epistasy of synthesis") or by competition with the corresponding endogenous gene transcript for trans-acting factors that are required for transcript stability or translation but are present in limiting concentration in the chloroplast [46]. The strategies to overcome this involve either replacement of the 5′ UTR of the endogenous gene with that from another photosynthetic gene [47] or, more elegantly, the development of synthetic variants of the 5′ UTR that are no longer subject to these limitations and therefore enable improved expression of the transgene [48]. Further studies into the design of synthetic promoters and UTRs, combined with improved knowledge of codon optimization rules, will advance the ability to engineer plastid metabolic pathways for customized functionalities and production efficiencies of commercial scale [49].

7. Regulation of RNA editing in chloroplasts

An important process of gene regulation is RNA editing. This occurs at posttranscriptional level through nucleotide modification for many functional genes. RNA editing restores the conserved amino acid residues for functional proteins in plants. Changes in RNA sequence of functional gene occurs during RNA editing, through the molecular mechanisms [50]. Cytidine-to-uridine editing and adenosine-to-inosine editing are two types of RNA editing identified in *Arabidopsis thaliana* [51]. RNA editing is a rare process where RNA polymerase is involved in insertion, deletion, and base substitution of nucleotide within the transcript [52–55]. Many studies reported the evidence of RNA editing in tRNA, rRNA, and mRNA. However, RNA editing has also been reported in noncoding RNA, like microRNAs of eukaryotes. The RNA editing occurs in all DNA-containing organelles like nucleus, mitochondria, and plastids. In nucleus, chloroplast and mitochondria RNA editing occurs during the process of transcription and posttranscriptional modifications [56, 57]. Caseinolytic protease complex component (CLPC1) plays a crucial role in RNA homeostasis [58]. Anyhow, discrete changes in RNA before its translation into protein occur by RNA editing. Besides this, RNA editing is also a vibrant mechanism to produce functional and molecular diversity [59].

In chloroplast gene expression system, RNA editing is an important posttranscriptional modification. The use of pentatricopeptide repeat (PPR) protein family for RNA editing in chloroplast has been reported [51]. Mostly genes in chloroplast are cotranscribed and arranged in clusters. To control gene expression, posttranscriptional RNA editing is an essential step, and this step is also required for gene function [52]. It has been studied that C-to-U editing is the major type of RNA editing in chloroplasts. In chloroplast, etioplast, and amyloplast of maize, expression of almost 15 different genes has been affected by 27 C-to-U RNA editing sites. In chloroplast, RNA editing plays an important role to correct harmful mutations instead of producing protein diversity. Genomic DNA sequence is not changed by C-to-U editing because this editing changes the nucleotide sequence only within RNA molecule. RNA polymerase is used to produce RNA editing [60]. Insertion, deletion, and base substitution are events of RNA editing. That is why RNA editing can reverse harmful genomic mutations in consistent RNA transcript. In chloroplast, different sites are edited by C-to-U RNA editing enzymes as well [61]. Around 126 C-to-U editing events and 11 U-to-C editing events were identified in the chloroplast DNA of moth orchid (*P. aphrodite* subsp. Formosana). In leaf tissues, 110 editing events and in floral tissue, 106 editing events were identified. In non-protein-coding RNA such as introns, tRNA, and regulatory sequences, RNA editing occurred [62]. Besides C-to-U editing, which is mostly reported in chloroplast of plants, adenosine-to-inosine editing in plastid tRNA of *Arabidopsis thaliana* has also been characterized. Adenosine-to-inosine editing was recognized in the anticodon of the plastid tRNA-Arg (ACG). AtTadA gene expression is involved in adenosine-to-inosine editing in the chloroplast [51].

8. Conclusions and future directions

Chloroplasts are the most important solar-energy-capturing natural systems on earth. They not only capture it but also convert it into a form useful for all living organism on earth. Molecular oxygen is liberated as a by-product, which is a vital source for respiration of all aerobic organisms. Chloroplasts are believed to be evolved from prokaryotic ancestors through a process known as endosymbiosis. Chloroplast contains circular genome having compactly arranged genes, which are involved in not only photosynthesis but also many other vital biological processes. Keeping in view its utmost physiological importance, plant as well as algal plastome has been engineered for a number of agronomic as well as pharmaceutical traits [63, 64]. Advancements in molecular biology and transgenic technology have further groomed importance of the organelle, and they are the most ideal ones for the expression of transgene. Resolving current limitations including vector design, gene regulation control and DNA delivery may further improve this important field of biotechnology [65]. Synthetic biology is being explored in this regard, which is expected to play a major role in enhancing contribution of chloroplasts not only for sustainable food production but also for other important molecules in future.

Author details

Muhammad Sarwar Khan, Ghulam Mustafa* and Faiz Ahmad Joyia

*Address all correspondence to: drmustafa8@gmail.com

Centre of Agricultural Biochemistry and Biotechnology (CABB), University of Agriculture, Faisalabad, Pakistan

References

[1] Borg S, Brinch-Pederson H, Tauvis B, Holm PB. Iron transport, deposition and bioavailability in the wheat and barley grain. Plant and Soil. 2009;**325**:15-24. DOI: 10.1007/s11104-009-0046-6

[2] Solymosi K, Bertrand M. Soil metals, chloroplasts, and secure crop production: A review. Agronomy for Sustainable Development. 2012;**32**:245-272. DOI: 10.1007/ s13593-011-0019-z

[3] Khan MS. Plastid genome engineering in plants: Present status and future trends. Molecular Plant Breeding. 2012;**3**:91-102

[4] Adem M, Beyene D, Feyissa T. Recent achievements obtained by chloroplast transformation. Plant Methods. 2017;**13**:30

[5] Khan MS. Plant biology: Engineered male sterility. Nature. 2005;**436**:783-785. DOI: 10.1038/ 436783a

[6] Richter LV, Yang H, Yazdani M, Hanson MR, Ahner BA. A downstream box fusion allows stable accumulation of a bacterial cellulase in *Chlamydomonas reinhardtii* chloroplasts. Biotechnology for Biofuels. 2018;**11**:133

[7] Bock R. Engineering plastid genomes: Methods, tools, and applications in basic research and biotechnology. Annual Review of Plant Biology. 2015;**66**:31-33. DOI: 10.1146/ annurev-arplant-050213-040212

[8] Michoux F, Ahmad N, Hennig A, Nixon PJ, Warzecha H. Production of leafy biomass using temporary immersion bioreactors: An alternative platform to express proteins in transplastomic plants with drastic phenotypes. Planta. 2013;**237**:903-908. DOI: 10.1007/ s00425-012-1829-1

[9] Khan MS, Khalid AM, Malik KA. Intein-mediated protein trans-plicing and transgene containment in plastids. Trends in Biotechnology. 2005;**23**:217-220

[10] Khan MS, Hameed W, Nozoe M, Shiina T. Disruption of the psbA gene by the copy correction mechanism reveals that the expression of plastid-encoded genes is regulated by photosynthesis activity. Journal of Plant Research. 2007;**120**:421-430

[11] Lin MT, Occhialini A, Andralojc PJ, Parry MA, Hanson MR. A faster RuBisCO with potential to increase photosynthesis in crops. Nature. 2014;**513**:547-550. DOI: 10.1038/nature13776

[12] Nazir S, Khan MS. Chloroplast-encoded chlB gene from *Pinus thunbergii* promotes root and early chlorophyll pigment development in *Nicotiana tabaccum*. Molecular Biology Reports. 2012;**39**:10637-10646. DOI: 10.1007/s11033-012-1953-9

[13] Khan MS. Engineering photorespiration in chloroplasts: A novel strategy for increasing biomass production. Trends in Biotechnology. 2007;**25**:437-440

[14] Jin S, Kanagaraj A, Verma D, Lange T, Daniell H. Release of hormones from conjugates: Chloroplast expression of βglucosidase results in elevated phytohormone levels with significant increase in biomass and protection from aphids and whiteflies conferred by sucrose esters. Plant Physiology. 2011;**155**:222-235. DOI: 10.1104/pp.110.160754

[15] Zhang J, Khan SA, Hasse C, Ruf S, Heckel DG, Bock R. Full crop protection from an insect pest by expression of long double-stranded RNAs in plastids. Science. 2015;**347**:991-994. DOI: 10.1126/science.1261680

[16] Jin S, Zhang X, Daniell H. Pinellia ternata agglutinin expression in chloroplasts confers broad spectrum resistance against aphid, whitefly, Lepidopteran insects, bacterial and viral pathogens. Plant Biotechnology Journal. 2012;**10**:313-327. DOI: 10.1111/j.1467-7652.2011.00663.x

[17] Chen P-J, Senthilkumar R, Jane W-N, He Y, Tian Z, Yeh K-W. Transplastomic Nicotiana benthamiana plants expressing multiple defence genes encoding protease inhibitors and chitinase display broad-spectrum resistance against insects, pathogens and abiotic stresses. Plant Biotechnology Journal. 2014;**12**:503-515. DOI: 10.1111/pbi.12157

[18] Lee SB, Kwon HB, Kwon SJ, Park SC, Jeong MJ, Han SE, et al. Accumulation of trehalose within transgenic chloroplasts confers drought tolerance. Molecular Breeding. 2003;**11**: 1-13. DOI: 10.1023/A:1022100404542

[19] Khan MS, Kanwal B, Nazir S. Metabolic engineering of the chloroplast genome reveals that the yeast *ArDH* gene confers enhanced tolerance to salinity and drought in plants. Frontiers in Plant Science. 2015;**6**:725. DOI: 10.3389/fpls.2015.00725

[20] Li K, Qiu H, Zhou M, Lin Y, Guo Z, Lu S. Chloroplast protein 12 expression alters growth and chilling tolerance in tropical forage *Stylosanthes guianensis* (Aublet) Sw. Frontiers in Plant Science. 2018;**9**:1319. DOI: 10.3389/fpls.2018.01319

[21] Narra M, Kota S, Velivela Y, Ellendula R, Allini VR, Abbagani S. Construction of chloroplast transformation vector and its functional evaluation in *Momordica charantia* L. 3 Biotech. 2018;**8**(3):140. DOI: 10.1007/s13205-018-1160-z

[22] Gan Q, Jiang J, Han X, Wang S, Lu Y. Engineering the chloroplast genome of oleaginous marine microalga *Nannochloropsis oceanica*. Frontiers in Plant Science. 2018;**9**:439. DOI: 10.3389/fpls.2018.00439

[23] Zienkiewicz M, Krupnik T, Drozak A, Golke A, Romanowska E. Transformation of the *Cyanidioschyzon merolae* chloroplast genome: Prospects for understanding chloroplast function in extreme environments. Plant Molecular Biology. 2016;**93**:171-183

[24] Stael S, Wurzinger B, Mair A, Mehlmer N, Vothknecht UC, Teige M. Plant organellar calcium signalling: An emerging field. Journal of Experimental Botany. 2012;**63**:1525-1542

[25] Rocha AG, Vothknecht UC. The role of calcium in chloroplasts: An intriguing and unresolved puzzle. Protoplasma. 2012;**249**:957-966

[26] Sai J, Johnson CH. Dark-stimulated calcium ion fluxes in the chloroplast stroma and cytosol. The Plant Cell. 2002;**14**:1279-1291

[27] Johnson CH, Knight MR, Kondo T, Masson P, Sedbrook J, Haley A, et al. Circadian oscillations of cytosolic and chloroplastic free calcium in plants. Science. 1995;**269**:1863-1865

[28] Nomura H, Komori T, Kobori M, Nakahira Y, Shiina T. Evidence for chloroplast control of external Ca^{2+}-induced cytosolic Ca^{2+} transients and stomatal closure. The Plant Journal. 2008;**53**:988-998

[29] Seigneurin-Berny D, Gravot A, Auroy P, Mazard C, Kraut A, Finazzi G, et al. HMA1, a new Cu-ATPase of the chloroplast envelope, is essential for growth under adverse light conditions. The Journal of Biological Chemistry. 2006;**281**:2882-2892

[30] Teardo E, Formentin E, Segalla A, Giacometti GM, Marin O, Zanetti M, et al. Dual localization of plant glutamate receptor AtGLR3.4 to plastids and plasma membrane. Biochimica et Biophysica Acta. 2011;**1807**:359-367

[31] Wilson ME, Jensen GS, Haswell ES. Two mechanosensitive channel homologs influence division ring placement in *Arabidopsis* chloroplasts. The Plant Cell. 2011;**23**:2939-2949

[32] Zimorski V, Ku C, Martin WF, Gould SB. Endosymbiotic theory for organelle origins. Current Opinion in Microbiology. 2014;**22**:38-48

[33] Bendich AJ. Circular chloroplast chromosomes: The grand illusion. The Plant Cell. 2004; **16**:1661-1666

[34] Hadariova L, Vesteg M, Hampl V, Krajcovic J. Reductive evolution of chloroplasts in non-photosynthetic plants, algae and protists. Current Genetics. 2018;**64**:365-387

[35] Del Cortona A, Leliaert F, Bogaert KA, Turmel M, Boedeker C, Janouškovec J, et al. The plastid genome in cladophorales green algae is encoded by hairpin chromosomes. Current Biology. 2017;**27**:3771-3782

[36] Wicke S, Schneeweiss GM, dePamphilis CW, Müller KF, Quandt D. The evolution of the plastid chromosome in land plants: Gene content, gene order, gene function. Plant Moleular Biology. 2011;**76**:273-297

[37] O'Neill BM, Mikkelson KL, Gutierrez NM, Cunningham JL, Wolff KL, Szyjka SJ, et al. An exogenous chloroplast genome for complex sequence manipulation in algae. Nucleic Acids Research. 2012;**40**:2782-2792

[38] Bertalan I, Munder MC, Weiß C, Kopf J, Fischer D, Johanningmeier U. A rapid, modular and marker-free chloroplast expression system for the green alga *Chlamydomonas reinhardtii*. Journal of Biotechnology. 2015;**195**:60-66

[39] Noor-Mohammadi S, Pourmir A, Johannes TW. Method to assemble and integrate biochemical pathways into the chloroplast genome of *Chlamydomonas reinhardtii*. Biotechnology and Bioengineering. 2012;**109**:2896-2903

[40] Oey M, Ross IL, Hankamer B. Gateway-assisted vector construction to facilitate expression of foreign proteins in the chloroplast of single celled algae. PLoS One. 2014;**9**:e86841

[41] Scharff LB, Bock R. Synthetic biology in plastids. The Plant Journal. 2014;**78**:783-798

[42] Gimpel JA, Nour-Eldin HH, Scranton MA, Li D, Mayfield SP. Refactoring the six gene photosystem II core in the chloroplast of the green algae *Chlamydomonas reinhardtii*. ACS Synthetic Biology. 2016;**5**:589-596

[43] Macedo-Osorio KS, Perez-Espana VH, Garibay-Orijel C, Guzman-Zapata D, Duran-Figueroa NV, Badillo-Corona JA. Intercistronic expression elements (IEE) from the chloroplast of *Chlamydomonas reinhardtii* can be used for the expression of foreign genes in synthetic operons. Plant Molecular Biology. 2018;**98**:303

[44] Rasala BA, Muto M, Sullivan J, Mayfield SP. Improved heterologous protein expression in the chloroplast of *Chlamydomonas reinhardtii* through promoter and 5′ untranslated region optimization. Plant Biotechnology Journal. 2011;**9**:674-683

[45] Coragliotti AT, Beligni MV, Franklin SE, Mayfield SP. Molecular factors affecting the accumulation of recombinant proteins in the *Chlamydomonas reinhardtii* chloroplast. Molecular Biotechnology. 2011;**48**:60-75

[46] Choquet Y, Wollman FA. Translational regulations as specific traits of chloroplast gene expression. FEBS Letters. 2002;**529**:39-42

[47] Gimpel JA, Hyun JS, Schoepp NG, Mayfield SP. Production of recombinant proteins in microalgae at pilot greenhouse scale. Biotechnology and Bioengineering. 2015;**112**:339-345

[48] Specht EA, Mayfield SP. Synthetic oligonucleotide libraries reveal novel regulatory elements in *Chlamydomonas* chloroplast mRNAs. ACS Synthetic Biology. 2013;**2**:34-46

[49] Zoschke R, Bock R. Chloroplast translation: Structural and functional organization, operational control, and regulation. The Plant Cell. 2018;**30**:745-770

[50] Chateigner-Boutin AL, Ramos-Vega M, Guevara-García A, Andrés C, De La Luz Gutiérrez-Nava M, Cantero A, et al. CLB19, a pentatricopeptide repeat protein required for editing of rpoA and clpP chloroplast transcripts. The Plant Journal. 2008;**56**:590-602. DOI: 10.1111/j.1365-313X.2008.03634.x

[51] Karcher D, Bock R. Identification of the chloroplast adenosine-to-inosine tRNA editing enzyme. RNA. 2009;**15**:1251-1257. DOI: 10.1261/rna.1600609

[52] Zoschke R, Qu Y, Zubo YO, Börner T, Schmitz-Linneweber C. Mutation of the pentatricopeptide repeat-SMR protein SVR7 impairs accumulation and translation of chloroplast

ATP synthase subunits in *Arabidopsis thaliana*. Journal of Plant Research. 2013;**126**: 403-414. DOI: 10.1007/s10265-012-0527-1

[53] Sugita M, Sugiura M. Regulation of gene expression in chloroplasts of higher plants. Plant Molecular Biology. 1996;**32**:315-326. DOI: 10.1007/BF00039388

[54] Peeters NM, Hanson MR. Transcript abundance supercedes editing efficiency as a factor in developmental variation of chloroplast gene expression. RNA. 2002;**8**:497-511. DOI: 10.1017/S1355838202029424

[55] Hegeman CE, Halter CP, Owens TG, Hanson MR. Expression of complementary RNA from chloroplast transgenes affects editing efficiency of transgene and endogenous chloroplast transcripts. Nucleic Acids Research. 2005;**33**:1454-1464. DOI: 10.1093/nar/gki286

[56] Hayes ML, Reed ML, Hegeman CE, Hanson MR. Sequence elements critical for efficient RNA editing of a tobacco chloroplast transcript in vivo and in vitro. Nucleic Acids Research. 2006;**34**:3742-3754. DOI: 10.1093/nar/gkl490

[57] Bock R. Sense from nonsense: How the genetic information of chloroplasts is altered by RNA editing. Biochimie. 2000;**82**:549-557. DOI: 10.1016/S0300-9084(00)00610-6

[58] Zhang S, Zhang H, Xia Y, Xiong L. The caseinolytic protease complex component CLPC1 in *Arabidopsis* maintains proteome and RNA homeostasis in chloroplasts. BMC Plant Biology. 2018;**18**:192. DOI: 10.1186/s12870-018-1396-0

[59] Hirose T, Kusumegi T, Tsudzuki T, Sugiura M. RNA editing sites in tobacco chloroplast transcripts: Editing as a possible regulator of chloroplast RNA polymerase activity. Molecular and General Genetics. 1999;**262**:462-467. DOI: 10.1007/s004380051106

[60] Robbins JC, Heller WP, Hanson MR. A comparative genomics approach identifies a PPR-DYW protein that is essential for C-to-U editing of the *Arabidopsis* chloroplast accD transcript. RNA. 2009;**15**:1142-1153. DOI: 10.1261/rna.1533909

[61] Hayes ML, Dang KN, Diaz MF, Mulligan RM. A conserved glutamate residue in the C-terminal deaminase domain of pentatricopeptide repeat proteins is required for RNA editing activity. Journal of Biological Chemistry. 2015;**290**:10136-10142. DOI: 10.1074/jbc.M114.631630

[62] Chen TC, Liu YC, Wang X, Wu CH, Huang CH, Chang CC. Whole plastid transcriptomes reveal abundant RNA editing sites and differential editing status in *Phalaenopsis aphrodite* subsp. formosana. Botanical Studies. 2017;**58**:38. DOI: 10.1186/s40529-017-0193-7

[63] Kwon YM, Kim KW, Choi TY, Kim SY, Kim JYH. Manipulation of the microalgal chloroplast by genetic engineering for biotechnological utilization as a green biofactory. World Journal of Microbiology and Biotechnology. 2018;**34**:183. DOI: 10.1007/s11274-018-2567-8

[64] Khan MS, Joyia FA. Biotechnology and GM Crops. In: Developing Sustainable Agriculture: A Case Study of Pakistan. USA: CRC Press Taylor & Francis; 2018. pp. 375-388

[65] Khan MS, Mustafa G, Nazir S, Joyia FA. Plant molecular biotechnology: Applications of transgenics. In: Applied Molecular Biotechnology: The Next Generation of Genetic Engineering. USA: CRC Press Taylor & Francis; 2016. pp. 61-89

Chapter 5

Understanding Plant Responses to Drought and Salt Stresses: Advances and Challenges in "Omics" Approaches

Mohammad Sayyar Khan and
Mudassar Nawaz Khan

Additional information is available at the end of the chapter

http://dx.doi.org/10.5772/intechopen.81041

Abstract

Global climatic changes and the temperature-associated fluctuations in drought, soil and water salinization and flooding have resulted in huge pressure on crop plants for their optimum yield potential. These challenges have to be met through innovative scientific technologies. Recent advances in the "Omics" approaches such as transcriptomics, proteomics and metabolomics offer new dimensions for understanding plant responses to drought and salt stresses and identification of major genes/QTLs for generation of resistant germplasm. Most importantly, the proteomics coupled with bioinformatics tools have accelerated the proteins characterization at the organ, tissue, organelle and membrane levels. Here we present an update on the progress of "Omics" approaches to understand plant responses to drought and salt stress particularly in the last decade. Future challenges and solution efforts are also discussed in the ways of omics approaches. The need for research involving integrated omics technologies with advanced tools and to meet the future challenges toward practical implementation of these technologies for crop improvement against drought and salinity stresses is also discussed.

Keywords: abiotic stresses, omics, proteomics, transcriptomics, mutants, map-based cloning

1. Introduction

Abiotic stresses, particularly drought, salt and low and high temperatures adversely affect plant growth and productivity and collectively account for more than 50% yield losses in important crop plants worldwide [1]. The resultant adverse changes in plant growth and productivity are orchestrated at the morphological, molecular and physiological levels [2]. The physiological effects of these stress conditions on plant developmental processes are mostly overlapping. Drought and salt stresses, in particular affect plants physiological and developmental processes by imposing osmotic and oxidative stresses. In addition, salt stress causes ionic stress and Na^+ toxicity. These stress conditions, in turn, induce cellular damages resulting in the disruption of ionic and osmotic [3]. In response to these stress conditions, plants generate a set of events comprising perception and transduction of stress signals. These changes ultimately result into expression of stress-related genes that induces alterations in metabolic processes [3]. The abiotic stress responses are generally polygenic in nature and are shared in multiple abiotic stresses [4].

Being a polygenic trait, achieving abiotic stress tolerance in crop plants through conventional breeding is a tedious and time-consuming approach. In this respect, comparative genomics has been utilized to explore candidate genes conferring tolerance to salt, drought and extreme temperature stresses in several plants [5, 6]. In recent years, appreciable work has been conducted to identify abiotic stress-related transcriptomes and proteomes in several plant species. The availability of these information in plants have paved the way for dissecting abiotic stress responses at the molecular level that provided a base for transgenic approaches against abiotic stresses. These approaches were utilized to engineer several crop plants in order to enhance their abiotic stress tolerance [4, 7]. However, taking into consideration the polygenic nature of abiotic stress tolerance, detailed transcriptomic and proteomic studies are required across the plant species to fully dissect the stress-response pathway. Such information will add to the current efforts to find suitable genes for plant transformation against abiotic stresses. The current review summarizes the recent findings on abiotic stress tolerance-related transcriptomic and proteomic studies in plant species.

2. Progress in functional and molecular genomics toward understanding stress perception

Abiotic stress tolerance is a polygenic trait that involves the expression of many sets of genes working in different pathways [8]. Plants have a well-organized system of sensing the environmental signals and responding to them in the form of gene expression [9]. The process of stress perception is comprised of a set of events including stress signaling, stress transduction and gene expression that result in accumulation of transcription factors, stress-related proteins, enzymes and metabolites (**Figure 1**). In order to fully understand the plants abiotic stress tolerance, and to modify it with the help of transgenic technologies, understanding the process of stress perception at the molecular level is very important. The application of functional genomics technologies has added new dimensions to our understanding of plant responses to environmental stresses [10]. The progress of abiotic stress tolerance in plants through conventional breeding programs has met with limited success, mainly because of the polygenic nature of abiotic stress responses in plants. However, during the last decade, considerable progress was made toward development of functional genomic tools that allowed the functional

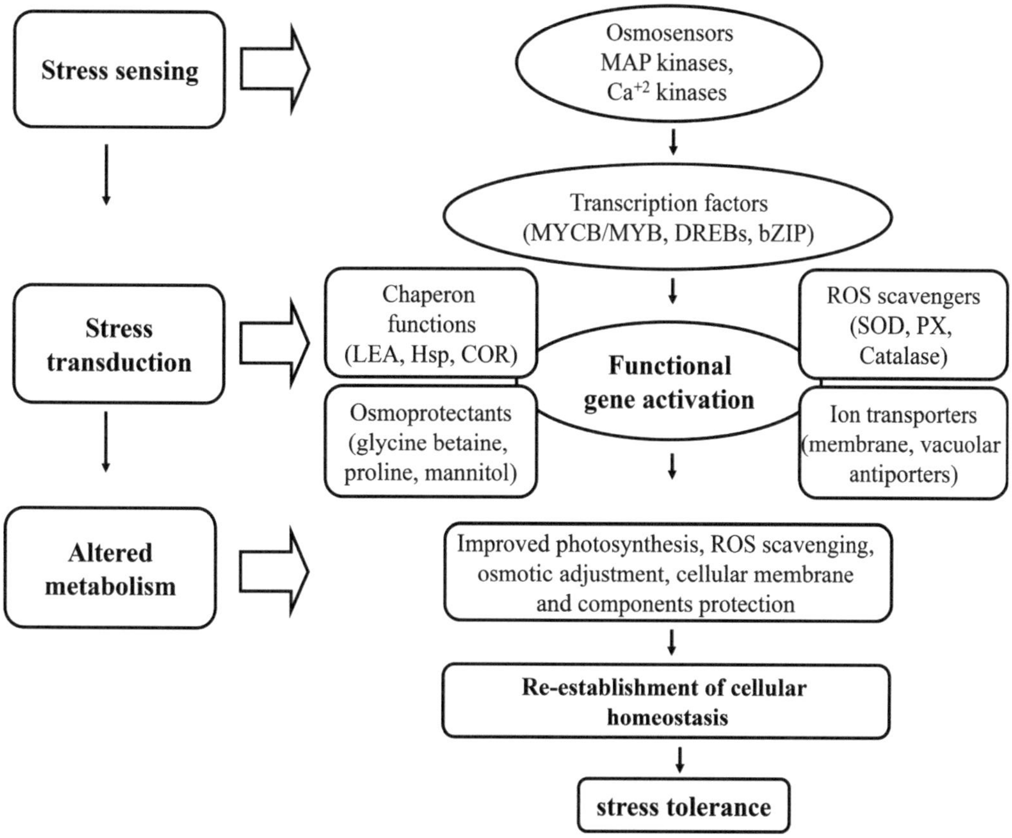

Figure 1. The process of plant response to abiotic stresses. The plant abiotic stress response pathway involves stress sensing, stress transduction and altered metabolism. Stress tolerance is achieved through expression of a large number of genes that accumulate stress-related transcription factors, chaperon function proteins, ROS scavenging enzymes, primary and secondary metabolites, osmoprotectants and cellular and vacuolar membrane antiporters.

dissection of the genetic determinants associated with abiotic stress responses. Major breakthroughs included (1) development of molecular markers for gene mapping and the construction of associated maps, (2) the development of expressed sequence tags (ESTs) libraries, (3) the complete sequencing of *Arabidopsis*, maize and rice genomes, (4) the development of T-DNA tagged mutagenic populations of *Arabidopsis* and (5) the development of forward genetics tools such as Targeting Induced Local Lesions in genomes (TILLING) technique to assess functional analysis of genes [11].

3. Map-based cloning of abiotic stress-related genes

Exploring genome sequences of *Arabidopsis* and rice and progress toward development of molecular markers and some new techniques has enabled positional cloning of mutated genes and natural alleles. A large number of molecular markers including single nucleotide polymorphisms (SNPs), simple sequence repeats (SSRs) and insertions/deletions (InDels) are available for *Arabidopsis* and rice plants. Map-based cloning approach that uses these various molecular markers have been used to identify a large number of abiotic stress-related genes such as the salt overly sensitive (*SOS1*, *SOS2*, *SOS3*, *SOS4* and *SOS5*) genes, and other stress-responsive genes [10]. For generation of mutant lines, ethyl methane sulfonate and irradiations have been extensively used so far. In addition, the recent development of new techniques such as stress-associated genes (SAGs) and TILLING have added new dimensions in identifying mutations in stress-related genes and variant alleles [12]. In the near future, these techniques will be available for a number of crop plants such as *Arabidopsis*, wheat, maize, rice and brassica [13].

Map-based cloning strategy has also been exploited to unravel abiotic stress-related QTLs in plants. As abiotic stress tolerance trait is polygenic in nature, the QTLs studies have received immense importance in understanding stress responses [14]. Recently, using map-based cloning, a large number of drought and salt stress-related QTLs have been reported in crop plants. QTLs were mapped in *Oryza sativa* for abiotic stress tolerance [15, 16], *Brassica napus* for salt tolerance [17], maize for salt tolerance [18], wheat for drought tolerance [19] and cotton for salt tolerance [20]. Gene stacking approach through marker-assisted selection was successfully used in an elite rice cultivar for stacked QTLs related to biotic and abiotic stresses (submergence and salinity tolerance) [21, 22]. Two out of 10 pyramid lines showed adequate tolerance to all tested stresses including abiotic stresses. Similar studies using abiotic stress tolerance genes/QTLs need to be extended to other crop plants.

4. Development of mutant populations

The use of mutant populations of plants, developed through insertional mutagenesis is an important tool to dissect the functions of abiotic stress-related genes [23]. Insertional mutagenesis is accomplished through T-DNA or transposable elements. Such mutant populations are available for *Arabidopsis* and rice plants. These saturation mutant populations of Arabidopsis and rice cover more than 90% of their genes that could be employed for characterization of abiotic stress tolerance genes [24]. Development of high throughput genomic platforms such as serial analysis of gene expression (SAGE), HRM (differential display, high resolution melt) analysis, TILLING, microarray, etc. have made rapid analysis of these mutation events. A large number of abiotic stress-related genes have been identified using *Arabidopsis* and rice knockout populations. In a 250,000 independent T-DNA insertional Arabidopsis population, more than 200 mutants were found with altered stress responses. Some of these include mutations in genes encoding transcription factors, ABA biosynthetic enzymes and sodium transporter high affinity K+ transporter (HKT1) [25]. Recent progress on the generation of T-DNA insertion lines have been reviewed in several articles [26, 27].

Along with T-DNA and transposable elements based mutant populations; the need for alternative means of studying gene function is growing day by day. This is mainly because of the low number of *Arabidopsis* and rice tagged genes that code for clear phenotypes [28]. Recently, traps and activation tagging have been focused as the alternative means of gene tagging [29, 30]. Trap and activation techniques have been widely used for generation of tagged populations of *Arabidopsis* and rice.

5. Transcriptomic analysis

Progress in transcriptomic analysis tools has revealed massive genomic sequence information in many plants. Identification of the partial or complete cDNAs sequences provide a holistic picture of the transcriptomes. The available ESTs are organized in three main databases, that is, NCBI, TIGR and Sputnik, which organize these ESTs with fully characterized gene sequences. Abiotic stress-related ESTs have contributed a great deal in exploring gene expression profiles of stress tolerance-related traits in in *Arabidopsis* and rice [31].

In recent years, different functional and molecular tools were used to identify abiotic stress-responsive genes in plants. These included genome wide physical and genetic mapping of chromosomes, isolation and sequencing of genes, ESTs, proteomics techniques and cDNA microarray analysis [32]. Particularly, the cDNA and microarrays were widely used to study gene expression profiles in Arabidopsis, potato, rice, sorghum, maize and wheat under abiotic stresses. The identified genes/proteins include late embryogenesis abundance (LEA) proteins, compatible osmolytes, ROS scavengers and proteins involved in signal transduction.

The genomic approaches related to abiotic stress tolerance in plants are summarized (**Table 1**). In one study, Oono et al. [33] used a full-length cDNA microarray containing 7000 *Arabidopsis* full-length cDNAs and identified 152 rehydration-inducible genes. Among the 152 rehydration-inducible genes, 58 genes showed proline- and hypoosmolarity-inducible gene expression. Similar study was conducted in Arabidopsis under drought stress [34]. Transcriptomic analysis of *M. sativa* and *M. esculenta* revealed expression of several genes responsive to salt and drought, respectively [35, 36]. In rice plants, the pioneering work came from Rabbani et al. [37]. They used cDNA and gel microarray analysis to identify cold, drought, salinity and ABA inducible genes. They identified 73 stress inducible genes, among which 15 genes were highly responsive to all four treatments. Lan et al. [38] determined and compared the drought and wounding stress-related gene expression profiles. Drought stress regulated many of the pollination/fertilization-related genes. Similarly, the drought stress-related transcriptomic analysis was conducted in some other studies in rice [39]. Using a cDNA microarray, 486 salt responsive ESTs were determined in shoots of rice plants under salt stress [40]. Moreover, Hmida-Sayari et al. [41] used the cDNA amplified fragment length polymorphism (AFLP) technique to investigate the expression profile of potato under salt stress. The expression profile showed 5000 bands, of which 154 were up-regulated, while 120 were down-regulated. Most of these ESTs were found to have a role in biotic and abiotic stresses. Sequence comparison of some of these fragments revealed close homologies with proteins, involved in cell wall structure, stress proteins such as glyceraldehyde dehydrogenase and proteins related to hypersensitive response to pathogens. Approximately 20,000 ESTs were generated from a cDNA library constructed

Species	Stress type	Findings	Reference
Arabidopsis thaliana	Drought	Total of 152 rehydration-inducible genes were identified.	Oono et al. [33]
A. thaliana	Drought	Translational regulation of 2000 genes was evaluated	Kawaguchi et al. [34]
Medicago sativa	Salt	Expression of large number of genes including 86 transcription factors was altered significantly	Postnikova et al. [35]
Manihot esculenta	Drought	Up-regulation of 1300 drought-responsive genes	Utsumi et al. [36]
Oryza sativa	Salt, drought	73 stress inducible genes were identified, among which 15 genes were highly responsive to salt, drought and cold stresses	Rabbani et al. [37]
Oryza sativa	Drought	53.8% and 21% of the pollination/fertilization-related genes were regulated by dehydration and wounding, respectively	Lan et al. [38]
Oryza sativa	Drought	—	—
Oryza sativa	Drought	589 genes were found responsive to drought	Gorantla et al. [14]
Oryza sativa	Drought	About 55% of genes differentially expressed in roots of rice under drought stress	Moumeni et al. [39]
Oryza sativa	Salt	486 salt responsive ESTs were determined in shoots	Chao et al. [40]
Oryza sativa	Drought, salt	Differential expression of large number of genes encoding transcription factors in stress sensitive and tolerant genotypes	Shankar et al. [47]
Solanum tuberosum	Salt	Six ADP-ribosylation factors like proteins were identified.	Kim et al. [110]
Solanum tuberosum	Salt	Expression profile showed 5000 ESTs, of which 154 were up-regulated, and 120 were down-regulated	Hmida-Sayari et al. [41]
Solanum tuberosum	Salt, heat, drought	1476 stress-related ESTs were found	Rensink et al. [42]
Solanum tuberosum	Salt, heat	3314 clones were identified as up- or down regulated	Rensink et al. [43]
Sorghum bicolor	Drought	333 genes responded to ABA, NaCl or osmotic stress	—
S. bicolor	Drought	775 genes were found differentially expressed in response to drought stress	Pratt et al. [44]
S. bicolor	Drought	Differential expression of genes involved in photosynthesis, carbon fixation, antioxidants in sensitive and tolerant genotypes	Fracasso et al. [49]
Triticum aestivum	Salt	Gene expression of 1811 genes was changed in response to salt stress	—
Triticum aestivum	Drought	3831 transcripts showed changes in expression in the drought-tolerant genotype	Li et al. [45]
Triticum aestivum	Drought	Large number of genes including 309 differentially expressed genes, responsive to drought stress were up-regulated	Ma et al. [48]
Zea mays	Water stress	79 genes in placenta and 56 genes in endosperm, were up- and down regulated, simultaneously	—

Species	Stress type	Findings	Reference
Zea mays	Drought	Differential expression levels of cell-wall related and transporter genes were found to contribute to drought tolerance	Zheng et al. [46]
Zea mays	Drought	A total of 619 genes and 126 transcripts were identified whose expression was altered by drought stress	Song et al. [50]

Table 1. Drought and salinity stress-responsive transcriptomic studies in various plant species.

from potato leaves and roots, which were subjected to salt, heat, cold and drought stresses [42, 43]. Some of these ESTs were found to have sequence similarities with abiotic stress-responsive genes in other plant species. Similar transcriptomic studies were conducted in some other plants such as sorghum [44], wheat [45], and maize [46] subjected to drought and salt stresses.

Recently, transcriptomic analysis through RNA sequencing has been proved to be a powerful tool for analysis of drought and salt stress-responsive genes. RNA-Seq uses next generation sequencing to reveal quantities of RNA in a given sample in real time. Examples of transcriptomic analysis through RNA-Seq have been reported in several crop plants subjected to drought and salt stresses. Shankar et al. [47] studied comparative transcriptomic analysis in drought sensitive and tolerant rice cultivars. A total of 801 and 507 transcripts were found differentially expressed in drought-tolerant (N22) and salt-tolerant (Pokkali) rice cultivars, respectively, under stress conditions. Overall, the study identified common and cultivar-specific stress-responsive transcripts. Ma et al. [48] conducted RNA-Seq analysis in wheat to study the drought-responsive transcriptomic changes during reproductive stages under field conditions. A total of 115,656 genes were detected and among these, 309 genes were found differentially expressed under drought at various developmental stages. Fracasso et al. [49] conducted transcriptomic analysis to study responses of drought sensitive and tolerant sorghum genotypes subjected to drought stress. Several genes such as those involved in photosynthesis, carbon fixation and antioxidants were found differentially expressed in the two genotypes under drought stress. Correlation in maize flowering time and drought stress was studied through RNA-seq and bioinformatics tools [50]. A total of 619 genes were identified, among which the expression of 126 transcripts was altered by drought stress. Among drought-responsive genes, the important transcripts included zinc finger and NAC domains. The study also identified 20 genes such as transcription factor *HY5*, *PRR37* and *CONSTANS* involved in flowering times.

The above-mentioned transcriptomic studies revealed that RNA-Seq analysis could be used as a very powerful tool not only to study stress-specific gene expression analysis but also to explore differences between stress sensitive and tolerant genotypes of crop plants.

6. Proteomic analysis

The study and characterization of the complete set of proteins in a cell, organ or organism at a given time is termed as proteomics [51]. Along transcriptomic studies, proteome analysis has contributed much to our understanding of the expression of stress-related genes in plants under abiotic stress. Proteomic studies on plant responses to salinity and drought stresses are being explored at large scale. Proteomic approaches have been applied at whole plant, organ and at subcellular levels to unravel the stress-response mechanism in plants. The prominent proteomic studies in plant species facing drought and salinity stresses are summarized (**Table 2**). Proteomic studies on sugar beet under drought stress identified that heat-shock proteins, nucleoside diphosphate kinase, RuBisCO, Cu-Zn superoxide dismutase (SOD) and 2-Cys-peroxiredoxin were highly induced [52]. Kim et al. [53] conducted proteomic analysis of maize subjected to drought stress and identified proteins involved in metabolism, photosynthesis and stress responses. Proteomic analysis of *Arabidopsis* under drought stress revealed that branched-chain amino acid amino transferase 3 protein and zinc finger transcription factor oxidative stress 2 proteins had a significant role in drought stress responses in the plants that over-expressed ethylene response factor AtERF019 [54].

Species	Stress	Proteomic changes	Plant organ/ organelle	Reference
Beta Vulgaris	Drought	79 proteins showed significant changes under drought. Important were RuBisCO and 11 others involved in redox regulation, oxidative stress, signal transduction and chaperone activities	Leaf	Hajheidari et al. [52]
Oryza sativa	Drought	Out of 12 proteins, 10 were up-regulated and 2 were down-regulated. These were mainly grouped as defense, energy, metabolism, cell structure and signal transduction proteins	Leaf sheath	Ali and Komatsu [116]
Triticum durum	Drought	Out of 36 significantly changed proteins, 12 were increased in abundance while 24 were decreased. RuBisCO large subunit, triose phosphate isomerase, thiol-specific antioxidant protein, phosphoglycerate kinase were increased	Leaf	Caruso et al. [58]
Helianthus annuus	Drought	Six proteins related to stress and carbon metabolism were found significantly up-regulated in leaves of drought stressed sunflower leaves.	Leaf	—
Glycine max	Drought	32 proteins changed in root. HSP 70, actin B and methionine synthase were differentially changed in the 3 organs	Root Hypocotyl Leaf	Mohammadi et al. [59]
Brassica napus	Drought	35 proteins in sensitive and 32 in tolerant line were differentially expressed. Six proteins in F1 hybrid were common to sensitive and tolerant lines	Root	Mohammadi et al. [60]
Oryza sativa	Drought	Out of 900 identified proteins, 38% were changed in abundance compared to non-treated. Pathogenesis-related, chitinases and redox proteins were increased while tubulins and transport-related proteins were decreased.	Root	Mirzaei et al. [61]
Vitis vinifera	Drought	Early responding proteins included photosynthesis, glycolysis, translation, antioxidant defense, while late-responding proteins included transport, photorespiration, antioxidants, amino acid and carbohydrate metabolism	Shoot	Cramer et al. [117]

Species	Stress	Proteomic changes	Plant organ/ organelle	Reference
Zea mays	Drought	Identified proteins were involved metabolism, stress response, photosynthesis, and protein modification	Leaves	Kim et al. [15]
Glycine max	Drought	643 proteins were significantly changed in soybean seedlings recovering from drought stress. Majority of these proteins belonged to stress, hormone metabolism, glycolysis and redox categories.	Root including hypocotyl	Khan and Komatsu [64]
Zea mays	Drought	Abundance of 68 proteins was changed. Out of these, 46 proteins were increased while 22 were decreased. Asparagine synthetase, alpha-galactosidase, fatty acid desaturase and plastid proteins were among the highly changed proteins	Leaf	Zhao et al. [118]
Brassica napus	Drought	Abundance of 138 proteins was differentially changed. Drought-responsive differentially abundant proteins were involved in signal transduction, photosynthesis and glutathione-ascorbate metabolism.	Leaf	Wang et al. [67]
Solanum lycopersicum	Drought	A total of 31 proteins were differentially changed in abundance under drought and 54 were changed during recovery phase. ABA accumulation pointed activation of chloroplast to nucleus signaling pathway	Leaf	Tamburino et al. [65]
Phaseolus vulgaris	Drought	Abundance of HSP-70 protein was highly changed. Protein synthesis, proteolysis and folding-related proteins increased in abundance	Stem	Zadražnik et al. [66]
Brassica napus	Drought	Among the 79 significant identified proteins, nitrogen assimilation, and ATP and redox Homeostasis were up-regulated in water savers cultivars; while photosynthesis, carbohydrate, RNA processing and stress related proteins were increased in water spender cultivars during water stress	Leaf	Urban et al. [68]
Glycine max	Salt	Under 100 mM salt stress, seven proteins were found to be up- or down-regulated. LEA, b-conglycinin, elicitor peptide three precursor, and basic/helix–loop–helix protein were up-regulated. While protease inhibitor, lectin, and stem 31-kDa glycoprotein precursor were down-regulated	Root Hypocotyl	Aghaei et al. [71]
Hordeum vulgare	Salt	ROS scavenging proteins were up-regulated in the tolerant genotype, while iron uptake proteins were up-regulated in the sensitive one	Root	Witzel et al. [73]
Nicotiana tabaccum	Salt	Total 18 proteins were differentially expressed under salt stress. Photosynthesis related proteins were up-regulated while defense-related proteins were down-regulated	Leaves	—
Solanum lycopersicum	Salt	Total 23 salt stress-responsive proteins belonging to six functional groups were identified	Root, Hypocotyl	Chen et al. [119]
Glycine max	Salt	Metabolism-related proteins were found up- and down-regulated in leaves, hypocotyls and roots under salt stress	Root, Hypocotyl	Sobhanian et al. [75]

Species	Stress	Proteomic changes	Plant organ/ organelle	Reference
Phoenix dactylifera	Salt, drought	The levels of ATP synthase alpha and beta subunits, RuBisCO, photosynthesis and ROS-related proteins were significantly changed under both stresses	Leaves	El Rabey et al. [120]
Triticum aestivum	Salt, Drought	Of the total 124 stress responsive proteins, 26.61% were induced by drought, included chaperonin, cys-peroxiredoxin, ethylene response, and elongation factor; while 23.38% were induced by salinity stress, included bowman-birk type protease inhibitor, calcineurin B-like protein, cyclophilin and RNA binding proteins	Seed	Kamal et al. [121]
Oryza sativa	Salt	In the two different cultivars, 104 and 102 proteins were significantly altered. Actin-7, tubulin alpha, V-type proton ATPase, SOD and pyruvate decarboxylase were among the observed salt-induced proteins	Root	Damaris et al. [80]
Avena sativa	Salt	From 30 differential protein spots, protein related to calvin cycle, adenosine-triphosphate regulation-related and 50S ribosomal proteins decreased while antioxidant enzymes abundance were increased.	Leaf	Bai et al. [78]
Triticum aestivum	Salt	Out of total of 121 proteins, ubiquitination-related proteins, transcription factors, pathogen-related proteins and anti-oxidant enzymes were increased for homeostasis	Root	Jiang et al. [122]

Table 2. Drought and salinity stress-related proteomic studies in various plant species.

In addition to the above-mentioned studies of proteomic analysis on the whole plant level, some notable studies have also focused the impact of drought and salinity stresses on organ-specific proteomic constituents. The metabolism-related proteins such as the isoflavone reductase, were observed as down-regulated which possibly played an important role in plant defense against various stresses [55]. Leaf-specific protein analysis in other plants identified drought-responsive proteins. These studies were conducted in rice [56], sunflower [57], wheat [58] and soybean [59, 60]. Root-specific proteome analysis was conducted in a number of crops under various drought stress, which identified a wide range of proteins including those involved in pathogenesis, transport and oxidation-reduction reactions. Prominent studies were conducted incanola (*Brassica napus*) [60], soybean [59] and rice [61]. Similar studies were conducted in rice [62] and wheat [63] subjected to salt stress, which identified changes more prominently in metabolism-related gene expression. Khan and Komatsu [64] performed proteomic analysis of soybean root including hypocotyl during recovery from drought stress and concluded that peroxidase and aldehyde dehydrogenase scavenge toxic reactive oxygen species and reduce the load of harmful aldehydes for helping the plant to recover. In tomato facing drought stress, chloroplast to nucleus signaling pathway in connection to abscisic acid (ABA) signaling network was activated [65]. In common bean stem, heat-shock protein 70 was highly increased in abundance suggesting its role in restoration of normal conformations of proteins for cellular homeostasis [66]. Proteomic analysis of maize leaves under drought stress revealed that ABA regulates the signaling pathways pertaining to oxidative phosphorylation, photosynthesis and glutathione metabolism. Phosphorylation of β carbonic anhydrase 1 imparted adaptation to drought stress in *Brassica napus* [67]. Proteomic analysis of rapeseeds under drought stress indicated that nitrogen assimilation, oxidative phosphorylation, redox homeostasis, energy, photosynthesis and stress-related proteins were raised in abundance in different cultivars [68].

Salinization of arable lands may result in up to 50% land loss by the year 2050 [69]. Proteomic techniques have been employed for analyzing salt stress responses in plants. In salt-tolerant and -sensitive potato cultivars, photosynthesis-related proteins were down-regulated; whereas osmotin-like proteins, heat-shock proteins and protein inhibitors were up-regulated [70, 71]. In soybean, β-conglycinin, elicitor peptide three precursor, late embryogenesis-abundant protein, and basic/helix-loop-helix protein, were up-regulated, suggesting soybean adaptation to salt stress; whereas protease inhibitor, lectin and stem, 31-kDa glycoprotein precursor were down-regulated, suggesting the weakening of plant defense system under the salinity stress [72]. Differentiation of salt stress-related proteins was evaluated in tolerant and sensitive barley genotypes [73]. Another study conducted on barley found expression of germin-like and pathogenesis-related proteins important for salt stress responses [74]. ATP production-related glyceraldehyde-3-phosphate was down-regulated in soybean under salt stress [75]. Cupin domain protein 3.1 was revealed in enhancing seed germination in rice under salt stress [76]. In barley, salt stress increased the abundance of proteins related to anti-oxidation, signal transduction, protein biosynthesis, ATP generation and photosynthesis [77]. Proteomic analysis of oat leaves under salt stress indicated decrease in abundance of calvin cycle-related and adenosine-triphosphate regulation-related proteins; whereas antioxidant enzymes level was increased [78]. Alterations in proteomic profiles were recorded in wheat cultivars under salt stress [63]. Kamal et al. [79] reported a decrease in ATP synthase and V-type proton ATPase subunits; whereas cytochrome b6-f, germin-like-protein, glutamine synthetase, fructose-bis-phosphatealdolase, S-adenosylmethionine synthase and carbonic anhydrase were gradually increased. Damaris et al. [80] reported induction of actin-7, tubulin alpha, V-type proton ATPase, SOD and pyruvate decarboxylase in salt-stressed wheat cultivars. Proteomic analysis of wheat roots indicated differential expression of a number of proteins such as transcription factors, proteins related to ubiquitination pathogenesis and antioxidant enzymes under salt stress [81]. All the above discussed studies show the importance of proteomics in unraveling the vital information about the plants responses to abiotic stresses such as drought and salinity stress responses.

7. Metabolomic analysis

Metabolomics is one of the most important "Omics" technologies that can be applied to different organisms with little or no modification. The term metabolomics was introduced by Nicholson et al. [82], and since then it has been utilized extensively in agricultural research [83, 84]. The metabolite profiling provides valuable information on the stress tolerance mechanisms and may be applied to bioengineer plants with improved stress tolerance. Metabolomics studies reveal information about compounds involved in acclimation to the stress, those which are by-products as a result of disruption of normal homeostasis and those involved in signal transduction in response to the stresses [85]. Due to involvement of metabolites in important life processes, the field of metabolic profiling could contribute significantly to the study of stress biology in plants. Both primary and secondary metabolites have been shown to play important roles in responses of plants to drought and salinity stresses. Primary metabolites such as sugars, amino acids and intermediates of Krebs cycle were found with important roles in photosynthetic dysfunction and osmotic readjustment. While, the secondary metabolites such as antioxidant scavengers, coenzymes and regulatory molecules responded to specific stress conditions. Both qualitative and quantitative studies of metabolites in response to abiotic stress are helpful in not only determining the phenotypic response of the plant and screening for stress tolerant lines but also reveal the genetic and biochemical mechanisms underlying the stress condition [86].

Drought and salt stresses affect the process of photosynthesis, affecting CO_2 diffusion leading to photorespiration and hydrogen peroxide production, causing cell damage [87]. Most recently, Rabara et al. [88] analyzed the metabolomics profile of tobacco and soybean roots and leaves facing dehydration stress. The study revealed highest tissue specific accumulation of 4-hydroxy-2-oxoglutaric acid in tobacco roots and coumestrol in soybean roots; indicating 4-hydroxy-2-oxoglutaric acid and coumestrol can be used as markers for drought stress. Metabolomic analysis of intense drought-stressed grapevine leaves was conducted to reveal induction of several metabolites [89]. Metabolomic profiling of *Arabidopsis* exposed to drought and heat stresses in combination revealed accumulation of sucrose, maltose and glucose [90]. In tolerant and sensitive thyme facing water stress, metabolomics analysis revealed differential changes in carbohydrates, amino acids, fatty acids and organic acids profiles [91]. Metabolites related to the mechanisms of osmotic adjustment, ROS scavenging, cellular components protection and membrane lipid showed significant changes. Metabolomic and proteomic analysis of xylem sap in maize under drought stress revealed a higher abundance of cationic peroxidases, which with the increase in phenylpropanoids may lead to a reduction in lignin biosynthesis in the xylem vessels and could induce cell wall stiffening [92]. Catola et al. [93] reported that trans-2-hexenal showed a significant increase in water-stressed and recovered leaves respect to the well-watered ones in pomegranate plants. This indicated a possible role of the oxylipin pathway in the response to water stress. Metabolites changes in rice grains during water-stressed and recovery indicated involvement in stress signaling pathways such as gamma-amino butyric acid (GABA) biosynthesis, sucrose metabolism and antioxidant defense [94]. Zhang et al. [95] reported that myo-inositol and proline had striking regulatory profiles in *Medicago* indicating involvement in drought tolerance. Metabolite profiling of hybrid poplar genotypes revealed that amino acids, the antioxidant phenolic compounds catechin and kaempferol, as well as the osmolytes raffinose and galactinol exhibited increased abundance under drought stress, whereas metabolites involved in photorespiration, redox regulation and carbon fixation showed decreased abundance under drought stress [96]. Concentrations of flavonoids, glycosides of kaempferol, quercetin and cyanidin were found in *Arabidopsis* during drought stress [97].

Salinity stress has been investigated at metabolite level to reveal the response mechanism. In salinity-stressed barley plants, cell division and root elongation was found associated with accumulation of amino acids, sugars and organic acids [98]. Chen and Hoehenwarter [99] reported that sucrose, fructose, glycolysis intermediates and amino acids levels were altered in *Arabidopsis* under salinity stress. Further, metabolite changes were found positively correlated with growth potential and salt tolerance in rice genotypes for allantoin and glutamine [100]. Meulebroek et al. [101] carried out metabolomic profiling of tomato carotenoid content under salt stress. The results revealed that metabolites had several roles at the fruit level in salinity response; however, 46 metabolites had ascribed a noticeable role in carotenoid metabolism as well. In barley, concentrations of most amino acids such as 4-hydroxy-proline, arginine, citrulline, glutamine, phenylalanine, proline and amines increased significantly in roots facing salinity stress [102]. Behr et al. [103] carried out metabolomics analysis in *Suaeda maritima* exposed to salinity stress. Results revealed increase in metabolites associated with osmotic stress and photorespiration; furthermore, alanine fermentation was enhanced. Oxidative stress produced by salinity in roots of *Salicornia herbacea* induced defense metabolites such as shikimic acid, vitamin K1 and indole-3-carboxylic acid that are generated as a result of defense mechanisms, to protect against ROS [104]. Metabolomic profiling studies revealed that sugars, sugar alcohols, proline, TCA cycle intermediates, histidine, glutathione and GABA were accumulated in *Arabidopsis thaliana* under salt stress [105, 106]. Production of signaling molecules such as serotonin and gentisic acid increased in salt-tolerant varieties indicating their importance as biomarker. Ferulic acid and vanillic acid were also produced in high levels. In the salt sensitive varieties, elevated levels of 4-hydroxycinnamic acid and 4-hydroxybenzoic acid were found in the leaves [19]. Epidermal bladder cells help in salt dumping, improved potassium retention in leaf mesophyll and space provision for storage of metabolites [107]. The above discussion revealed that metabolomics is very important tool in investigating abiotic stress-response mechanisms such as those observed in drought and salt stresses.

8. The way forward

RNA-Seq and genome sequencing and proteomic techniques/technologies (2D, iTRAQ, MALDI, gel-free, label-free, LC-MS/MS-based technologies) have widened the dimensions of analyzing plant responses to abiotic stresses such as drought and salinity. Recent advances in the omics technologies have contributed considerably to our understanding of the plant abiotic stress-responsive mechanisms. In addition to advancing research in other related areas, emphasis has been on the proteomic analysis specific to whole plants, individual organs, tissues and cells [55]. These technologies are helping to characterize individual proteins specific to different organs, tissues and cells subjected to various abiotic stresses. Advanced proteomic information, coupled with other omics approaches would further strengthen the efforts to develop breeding programs based on identification of novel proteins/genes and their integration through marker-assisted selection. However, further efforts are required to focus on individual target points associated with "Omics" technologies and their application to dissect stress-responsive mechanisms. Research needs to be focused on several fronts such as more studies that target post translational modifications (PTMs), cell type-specific proteome analysis, advanced mapping populations in crop plants and comparative proteomic studies. PTMs of proteins may change their stability, subcellular localization, interactions with other proteins and ultimately proteins functioning. A number of studies revealed the important role of PTMs in protein functioning. Studies have been conducted to analyses protein phosphorylation in maize

[108, 109], phosphorylation and ubiquitination in *Arabidopsis* [110, 111] and glycosylation in soybean [112] under various abiotic stresses. In addition to improved methodologies, identification of more PTMs would unravel functional characterization of important proteins involved in stress-responsive mechanisms and plant adaptation to various abiotic stresses.

Individual proteins characterization and quantification is essential to fully explore the stress-responsive mechanisms in organs, tissues and cells. However, problems may arise due to the conventional methodologies such as protein detection on 2-DE gels [55]. Improved extraction methodologies may overcome such problems. Poor proteome coverage may be the result while detecting leaf proteome with abundance of RuBisCO that constitutes almost half of the total leaf proteins. However, proteome coverage may be improved with the recently adopted fractionation of crude protein extract. Similarly, quantification of stress responsive low abundance target proteins may be improved through selected reaction monitoring (SRM) technique [113, 114]. Such improved techniques would also help unravel commonly expressed proteins in different organs under multiple abiotic stresses. These advanced techniques coupled with improved bioinformatics approaches may help shed further light on plant responses to abiotic stresses. Recently, transgenic plants conferring abiotic stress tolerance have entered vigorous evaluations under greenhouse and filed conditions. Comparative proteomic studies of these transgenic plants may be helpful to characterize key stress-responsive factors among large number of commonly expressed proteins. Identification of major stress-responsive proteins coupled with advances in transcriptomics, metabolomics and bioinformatics tools would help unravel the complex interactions among stress-responsive signaling pathways. Moreover, omics approaches such as proteomics can be extremely helpful in analyzing post-stress recovery responses in the plants, revealing the key proteins/genes involved in the recovery stage [115].

9. Conclusions

Different omics tools have been exploited to unravel plant responses to drought and salt stresses. However, further studies should be conducted to integrate multiple omics approaches including phenomics coupled with RNA-Seq and state-of-the-art proteomic technologies. These future developments will provide further impetus to the ongoing efforts of developing drought- and salt-tolerant plants with comparatively improved growth and yield potential under realistic field conditions.

Author details

Mohammad Sayyar Khan* and Mudassar Nawaz Khan

*Address all correspondence to: sayyarkhankazi@aup.edu.pk

Genomics and Bioinformatics Laboratory, Faculty of Crop Production Sciences, Institute of Biotechnology and Genetic Engineering (IBGE), The University of Agriculture, Peshawar, Khyber Pakhtunkhwa, Pakistan

References

[1] Vahdati K, Leslie C. Abiotic Stress-Plant Responses and Applications in Agriculture. Rijeka, Croatia: In Tech; 2013

[2] Fraire-Velázquez S, Balderas-Hernández VE. Abiotic stress in plants and metabolic responses. In: Vahdati K, Leslie C, editors. Abiotic Stress-Plant Responses and Applications in Agriculture. Rijeka, Croatia: In Tech; 2013. DOI: 10.5772/45842

[3] Ruan CJ, Teixeira da Silva JA. Metabolomics: Creating new potentials for unraveling the mechanisms in response to salt and drought stress and for the biotechnological improvement of xero-halophytes. Critical Reviews in Biotechnology. 2011;**31**:153-169

[4] Peleg Z, Apse MP, Blumwald E. Engineering salinity and water stress tolerance in crop plants: Getting closer to the field. Advances in Botanical Research. 2011;**57**:406-432

[5] Gorantla M, Babu PR, Lachagari VBR, Reddy AMM, Wusirika R, Bennetzen JL, et al. Identification of stress-responsive genes in an indica rice (*Oryza sativa* L.) using ESTs generated from drought-stressed seedlings. Journal of Experimental Botany. 2007;**58**:253-265

[6] Delano-Frier JP, Aviles-Arnaut H, Casarrubias-Castillo K, Casique-Arroyo G, Castrillon-Arbelaez PA, Herrera-Estrella L, et al. Transcriptomic analysis of grain amaranth (*Amaranthus hypochondriacus*) using 454 pyrosequencing: Comparison with *A. tuberculatus*, expression profiling in stems and in response to biotic and abiotic stress. BMC Genomics. 2011;**12**:363

[7] Blumwald E. Engineering salt tolerance in plants. Biotechnology & Genetic Engineering Reviews. 2003;**20**:261-275

[8] Zhang J, Klueva NY, Wang Z, Wu R, Ho THD, Nguyen HT. Genetic engineering for abiotic stress resistance in crop plants. In Vitro Cellular & Developmental Biology. Plant. 2000;**36**:108-114

[9] Shinozaki K, Yamaguchi-Shinozaki K. Gene expression and signal transduction in water-stress response. Plant Physiology. 1997;**115**:327-334

[10] Vij S, Tyagi AK. Emerging trends in the functional genomics of the abiotic stress response in crop plants. Plant Biotechnology Journal. 2007;**5**:361-380

[11] Colbert T, Till BJ, Tompa R, Reynolds S, Steine MN, Yeung AT, et al. High-throughput screening for induced point mutations. Plant Physiology. 2001;**126**:480-484

[12] Henikoff S, Comai L. Single-nucleotide mutations for plant functional genomics. Annual Review of Plant Biology. 2003;**54**:375-401

[13] Wu JL, Wu C, Lei C, Baraoidan M, Bordeos A, Madamba MR, et al. Chemical- and irradiation-induced mutants of *indica* rice IR64 for forward and reverse genetics. Plant Molecular Biology. 2005;**59**:85-97

[14] Gorantla M, Babu PR, Reddy Lachagari VB, Feltus FA, Paterson AH, Reddy AR. Functional genomics of drought stress response in rice: Transcript mapping of annotated unigenes of an *indica*rice (*Oryza sativa* L. cv. Nagina 22). Current Science. 2005;**89**:496-514

[15] Gao JP, Lin HX. QTL analysis and map-based cloning of salt tolerance gene in rice. Methods in Molecular Biology. 2013;**956**:69-82

[16] Tiwari S, Krishnamurthi SL, Kumar V, Singh B, Rao AR, et al. Mapping QTLs for salt tolerance in rice (*Oryza sativa* L.) by bulked segregant analysis of recombinant inbred lines using 50K SNP chip. PLoS One. 2017;**11**(3):e0151076. DOI: 10.1371/journal.pone.0153610

[17] Lang L, Xu A, Ding J, Zhang Y, Zhao N, et al. Quantitative trait locus mapping of salt tolerance and identification of salt-tolerant genes in *Brassica napus* L. Frontiers in Plant Science. 2014;**8**:1000. DOI: 10.3389/fpls.2017.01000. eCollection 2017

[18] Luo M, Zhao Y, Zhang R, Xing J, Duan M, et al. Mapping of a major QTL for salt tolerance of mature field-grown maize plants based on SNP markers. BMC Plant Biology. 2017;**17**:140

[19] Gupta P, De B. Metabolomics analysis of rice responses to salinity stress revealed elevation of serotonin, and gentisic acid levels in leaves of tolerant varieties. Plant Signaling & Behavior. 2017;**12**:e1335845. DOI: 10.1080/15592324.2017.1335845

[20] Du L, Cai C, Wu S, Zhang F, Hou S, Guo W. Evaluation and exploration of favorable QTL alleles for salt stress related traits in cotton cultivars (*G. hirsutum* L.). PLoS One. 2016;**11** (3):e0151076. DOI: 10.1371/journal.pone.0151076

[21] Das G, Rao GJN. Molecular marker gene stacking for biotic and abiotic stress resistance genes in an elite rice cultivar. Frontiers in Plant Science. 2015;**6**:698

[22] Das G, Patra JK, Baek KH. Insight into MAS: A molecular tool for development of stress resistant and quality of rice through gene stacking. Frontiers in Plant Science. 2017;**8**:985

[23] Papdi C, Leung J, Joseph M. Genetic screens to identify plant stress genes. Methods in Molecular Biology. 2010;**639**:121-139

[24] Punjabi-Sabharwal V, Karan R, Khan T, Pareek A. Abiotic stress responses: Complexities in gene expression. In: Pareek A, Sopory SK, Bonhert HJ, Govindji, editors. Abiotic Stress Adaptation in Plants: Physiological, Molecular and Genomic Foundation. Springer Netherlands: Springer Dordrecht; 2010. pp. 177-198

[25] Koiwa H, Bressan RA, Hasegawa PM. Identification of plant stress-responsive determinants in *Arabidopsis* by large scale forward genetic screens. Journal of Experimental Botany. 2006;**57**:1119-1128

[26] Qu LJ, Qin G. Generation and characterization of Arabidopsis T-DNA insertion mutants. Methods in Molecular Biology. 2014;**1062**:241-258

[27] Prasanna S, Jain SM. Mutant resources and mutagenomics in crop plants. Emirates Journal of Food and Agriculture. 2017;**29**:651-657. DOI: 10.9755/ejfa.2017.v29.i9.86

[28] An G, Lee S, Kim SH, Kim SR. Molecular genetics using T-DNA in rice. Plant & Cell Physiology. 2005b;**46**:14-22

[29] Jiang SY, Ramachandran S. Natural and artificial mutants as valuable resources for functional genomics and molecular breeding. International Journal of Biological Sciences. 2010;**6**:228-251

[30] Springer PS. Gene traps, tools for plant development and genomics. The Plant Cell. 2000; **12**:1007-1020

[31] Rensink WA, Buell CR. Microarray expression profiling resources for plant genomics. Trends in Plant Science. 2005;**10**:603-609

[32] Abbasi FM, Komatsu S. A proteomic approach to analyze salt-responsive proteins in rice leaf sheath. Proteomics. 2004;**4**:2072-2081

[33] Oono Y, Seki M, Nanjo T, Narusaka M, Fujita M, Satoh R, et al. Monitoring expression profiles of *Arabidopsis* gene expression during rehydration process after dehydration using ca. 7,000 full-length cDNA microarray. The Plant Journal. 2003;**34**:868-887

[34] Kawaguchi R, Girke T, Bray EA, Bailey-Serres J. Differential mRNA translation contributes to gene regulation under non-stress and dehydration stress conditions in *Arabidopsis thaliana*. The Plant Journal. 2004;**38**:823-839

[35] Postnikova OA, Shao J, Nemchinov LG. Analysis of the alfalfa root transcriptome in response to salinity stress. Plant & Cell Physiology. 2013;**54**:1041-1055

[36] Utsumi Y, Tanaka M, Morosawa T, Kurotani A, Yoshida T, Mochida K, et al. Transcriptome analysis using a high-density oligomicroarray under drought stress in various genotypes of cassava: An important tropical crop. DNA Research. 2012;**19**:335-345

[37] Rabbani MA, Maruyama K, Abe H, Khan MA, Katsura K, Ito Y, et al. Monitoring expression profiles of rice genes under cold, drought, and high-salinity stresses and abscisic acid application using cDNA microarray and RNA gel-blot analyses. Plant Physiology. 2003; **133**:1755-1767

[38] Lan L, Li M, Lai Y, Xu Y, Kong Z, Ying K, et al. Microarray analysis reveals similarities and variations in genetic programs controlling pollination/fertilization and stress responses in rice (*Oryza sativa.*). Plant Molecular Biology. 2005;**59**:151-164

[39] Moumeni A, Satoh K, Kondoh H, Asano T, Hosaka A, Venuprasad R, et al. Comparative analysis of root transcriptome profiles of two pairs of drought-tolerant and susceptible rice near-isogenic lines under different drought stresses. BMC Plant Biology. 2011;**11**:174

[40] Chao DY, Luo YH, Shi M, Luo D, Lin HX. Salt-responsive genes in rice revealed by cDNA microarray analysis. Cell Research. 2005;**15**:796-810

[41] Hmida-Sayari A, Costa A, Leone A, Jaoua S, Gargouri-Bouzid R. Identification of salt stress-induced transcripts in potato leaves by cDNA-AFLP. Molecular Biotechnology. 2005;**30**:31-40

[42] Rensink W, Hart A, Liu J, Ouyang S, Zismann V, Buell CR. Analyzing the potato abiotic stress transcriptome using expressed sequence tags. Genome. 2005a;**48**:598-605

[43] Rensink WA, Iobst S, Hart A, Stegalkina S, Liu J, Buell CR. Gene expression profiling of potato responses to cold, heat, and salt stress. Functional & Integrative Genomics. 2005b; **5**:201-207

[44] Pratt LH, Liang C, Shah M, Sun F, Wang H, Reid SP, et al. Sorghum expressed sequence tags identify signature genes for drought, pathogenesis, and skotomorphogenesis from a milestone set of 16,801 unique transcripts. Plant Physiology. 2005;**139**:869-884

[45] Li YC, Meng FR, Zhang CY, Zhang N, Sun MS, Ren JP, et al. Comparative analysis of water stress-responsive transcriptomes in drought-susceptible and -tolerant wheat (*Triticum aestivum* L.). Journal of Plant Biology. 2012;**55**:349-360

[46] Zheng J, Fu J, Gou M, Huai J, Liu Y, Jian M, et al. Genome-wide transcriptome analysis of two maize inbred lines under drought stress. Plant Molecular Biology. 2010;**72**:407-421

[47] Shankar R, Bhattacharjee A, Jain M. Transcriptome analysis in different rice cultivars provides novel insights into desiccation and salinity stress responses. Scientific Reports. 2016;**6**:23719. DOI: 10.1038/srep23719

[48] Ma J, Li R, Wang H, Li D, Wang X, Zhang Y, et al. Transcriptomics analyses reveal wheat responses to drought stress during reproductive stages under field conditions. Frontiers in Plant Science. 2017;**8**:592. DOI: 10.3389/fpls.2017.00592

[49] Fracasso A, Trindade LM, Amaducci M. Drought stress tolerance strategies revealed by RNA-Seq in two sorghum genotypes with contrasting WUE. BMC Plant Biology. 2016; **16**:115

[50] Song K, Kim HC, Shin S, Kim KH, Moon JC, Kim JY, et al. Transcriptome analysis of flowering time genes under drought stress in maize leaves. Frontiers in Plant Science. 2017;**8**:267

[51] Wilkins MR, Sanchez JC, Gooley AA, Appel RD, Humphery-Smith I, Hochstrasser DF, et al. Progress with proteome projects: Why all proteins expressed by a genome should be identified and how to do it. Biotechnology & Genetic Engineering Reviews. 1996;**13**: 19-50

[52] Hajheidari M, Noghabi MA, Askari H, Heidari M, Sadeghian SY, Ober ES, et al. Proteome analysis of sugar beet leaves under drought stress. Proteomics. 2005;**5**:950-960

[53] Kim SG, Lee JS, Kim JT, Kwon YS, Bae DW, Bae HH, et al. Physiological and proteomic analysis of the response to drought stress in an inbred Korean maize line. Plant Omics. 2015;**8**:159-168

[54] Scarpeci TE, Frea VS, Zanor ML, Valle EM. Overexpression of AtERF019 delays plant growth and senescence, and improved drought tolerance in Arabidopsis. Journal of Experimental Botany. 2017;**68**:673-685

[55] Komatsu S, Hossain Z. Organ-specific proteome analysis for identification of abiotic stress response mechanism in crop. Frontiers in Plant Science. 2013;**4**:71. DOI: 10.3389/fpls.2013.00071

[56] Ke Y, Han G, He H, Li J. Differential regulation of proteins and phosphoproteins in rice under drought stress. Biochemical and Biophysical Research Communications. 2013;**379**:133-138

[57] Castillejo MA, Maldonado AM, Ogueta S, Jorrín JV. Proteomic analysis of responses to drought stress in sunflower (*Helianthus annuus*) leaves by 2DE gel electrophoresis and mass spectrometry. The Open Proteomics Journal. 2008;**1**:59-71

[58] Caruso G, Cavaliere C, Foglia P, Gubbiotti R, Samperi R, Laganà A. Analysis of drought responsive proteins in wheat (*Triticum durum*) by 2D-PAGE and MALDI-TOF mass spectrometry. Plant Science. 2009;**177**:570-576

[59] Mohammadi PP, Moieni A, Hiraga S, Komatsu S. Organ-specific proteomic analysis of drought-stressed soybean seedlings. Journal of Proteomics. 2012a;**75**:1906-1923

[60] Mohammadi PP, Moieni A, Komatsu S. Comparative proteome analysis of drought-sensitive and drought-tolerant rapeseed roots and their hybrid F1 line under drought stress. Amino Acids. 2012b;**43**:2137-2152

[61] Mirzaei M, Soltani N, Sarhadi E, Pascovici D, Keighley T, Salekdeh GH, et al. Shotgun proteomic analysis of long-distance drought signaling in rice roots. Journal of Proteome Research. 2012;**11**:348-358

[62] Liu CW, Hsu YK, Cheng YH, Yen HC, Wu YP, Wang CS, et al. Proteomic analysis of salt-responsive ubiquitin-related proteins in rice roots. Rapid Communications in Mass Spectrometry. 2012;**26**:1649-1660

[63] Guo G, Ge P, Ma C, Li X, Lv D, Wang S, et al. Comparative proteomic analysis of salt response proteins in seedling roots of two wheat varieties. Journal of Proteomics. 2012;**75**:1867-1885

[64] Khan MN, Komatsu S. Proteomic analysis of soybean root including hypocotyl during recovery from drought stress. Journal of Proteomics. 2016;**144**:39-50

[65] Tamburino R, Vitale M, Ruggiero A, Sassi M, Sannino L, Arena S, et al. Chloroplast proteome response to drought stress and recovery in tomato (*Solanum lycopersicum* L.). BMC Plant Biology. 2017;**17**:40

[66] Zadražnik T, Egge-Jacobsen W, Meglič V, Šuštar-Vozlič J. Proteomic analysis of common bean stem under drought stress using in-gel stable isotope labeling. Journal of Plant Physiology. 2017;**209**:42-50

[67] Wang L, Jin X, Li Q, Wang X, Li Z, Wu X. Comparative proteomics reveals that phosphorylation of β carbonic anhydrase 1 might be important for adaptation to drought stress in *Brassica napus*. Scientific Reports. 2016;**6**

[68] Urban MO, Vašek J, Klíma M, Krtková J, Kosová K, Prášil IT, et al. Proteomic and physiological approach reveals drought-induced changes in rapeseeds: Water-saver and water-spender strategy. Journal of Proteomics. 2017;**152**:188-205

[69] Ma H, Yang R, Song L, Yang Y, Wang Q, Wang Z, et al. Differential proteomic analysis of salt stress response in jute (Corchoruscapsularis&olitorius L.) seedling roots. Pakistan Journal of Botany. 2015;**47**:385-396

[70] Aghaei K, Ehsanpour AA, Komatsu S. Proteome analysis of potato under salt stress. Journal of Proteome Research. 2008a;**7**:4858-4868

[71] Aghaei K, Ehsanpour AA, Komatsu S. Potato responds to salt stress by increased activity of antioxidant enzymes. Journal of Integrative Plant Biology. 2009;**51**:1095-1103

[72] Aghaei K, Ehsanpour AA, Shah AH, Komatsu S. Proteome analysis of soybean hypocotyls and root under salt stress. Amino Acids. 2008b;**36**:91-98

[73] Witzel K, Weidner A, Surabhi GK, Borner A, Mock HP. Salt stress-induced alterations in the root proteome of barley genotypes with contrasting response towards salinity. Journal of Experimental Botany. 2009;**60**:3545-3557

[74] Witzel K, Matros A, Strickert M, Kaspar S, Peukert M, Mühling KH, et al. Salinity stress in roots of contrasting barley genotypes reveals time-distinct and genotype-specific patterns for defined proteins. Molecular Plant. 2014;**7**:336-355

[75] Sobhanian H, Razavizadeh R, Nanjo Y, Ehsanpour AA, Jazii FR, Motamed N, et al. Proteome analysis of soybean leaves, hypocotyls and roots under salt stress. Proteome Science. 2010;**8**:19

[76] Xu E, Chen M, He H, Zhan C, Cheng Y, Zhang H, et al. Proteomic analysis reveals proteins involved in seed imbibition under salt stress in rice. Frontiers in Plant Science. 2016;**7**:2006

[77] Rasoulnia A, Bihamta MR, Peyghambari SA, Alizadeh H, Rahnama A. Proteomic response of barley leaves to salinity. Molecular Biology Reports. 2011;**38**:5055-5063

[78] Bai J, Qin Y, Liu J, Wang Y, Sa R, Zhang N, et al. Proteomic response of oat leaves to long-term salinity stress. Environmental Science and Pollution Research. 2016:1-3

[79] Kamal AH, Cho K, Kim DE, Uozumi N, Chung KY, Lee SY, et al. Changes in physiology and protein abundance in salt-stressed wheat chloroplasts. Molecular Biology Reports. 2012;**39**:9059-9074

[80] Damaris RN, Li M, Liu Y, Chen X, Murage H, Yang P. A proteomic analysis of salt stress response in seedlings of two African rice cultivars. Biochimica et Biophysica Acta (BBA)-Proteins Proteomics. 2016;**1864**:1570-1578

[81] Jiang Q, Li X, Niu F, Sun X, Hu Z, Zhang H. iTRAQ-based quantitative proteomic analysis of wheat roots in response to salt stress. Proteomics. 2010;**17**. DOI: 10.1002/pmic.201600265

[82] Nicholson JK, Lindon JC, Holmes E. 'Metabonomics': Understanding the metabolic responses of living systems to pathophysiological stimuli via multivariate statistical analysis of biological NMR spectroscopic data. Xenobiotica. 1999;**29**:1181-1189

[83] Hagel JM, Mandal R, Han B, Han J, Dinsmore DR, Borchers CH, et al. Metabolome analysis of 20 taxonomically related benzylisoquinoline alkaloid-producing plants. BMC Plant Biology. 2015;**15**:220

[84] Misra BB, Yin Z, Geng S, de Armas E, Chen S. Metabolomic responses of arabidopsis suspension cells to bicarbonate under light and dark conditions. Scientific Reports. 2016;**6**

[85] Shulaeva V, Cortesa D, Miller G, Mittler R. Metabolomics for plant stress response. Physiologia Plantarum. 2008;**132**:199-208

[86] Hong J, Yang L, Zhang D, Shi J. Plant metabolomics: An indispensable system biology tool for plant science. International Journal of Molecular Sciences. 2016;**17**:767

[87] Hossain Z, López-Climent MF, Arbona V, Pérez-Clemente RM, Gómez-Cadenas A. Modulation of the antioxidant system in citrus under water logging and subsequent drainage. Journal of Plant Physiology. 2009;**166**:1391-1404

[88] Rabara RC, Tripathi P, Rushton PJ. Comparative metabolome profile between tobacco and soybean grown under water-stressed conditions. BioMed Research International. 2017;**2017**. ID 3065251. DOI: 10.1155/2017/3065251

[89] Griesser M, Weingart G, Schoedl-Hummel K, Neumann N, Becker M, Varmuza K, et al. Severe drought stress is affecting selected primary metabolites, polyphenols, and volatile metabolites in grapevine leaves (*Vitis vinifera* cv. Pinot noir). Plant Physiology and Biochemistry. 2015;**88**:17-26

[90] Rizhsky L, Liang H, Shuman J, Shulaev V, Davletova S, Mittler R. When defense pathways collide.The response of Arabidopsis to a combination of drought and heat stress. Plant Physiology. 2004;**134**:1683-1696

[91] Moradi P, Ford-lloyd B, Pritchard J. Metabolomic approach reveals the biochemical mechanisms underlying drought stress tolerance in thyme. Analytical Biochemistry. 2017;**527**:49-62

[92] Alvarez S, Marsh EL, Schroeder SG, Schachtman DP. Metabolomic and proteomic changes in the xylem sap of maize under drought. Plant, Cell & Environment. 2008;**31**:325-340

[93] Catola S, Marino G, Emiliani G, Huseynova T, Musayev M, Akparov Z, et al. Physiological and metabolomic analysis of Punicagranatum (L.) under drought stress. Planta. 2016; **243**:441-449

[94] Nam KH, Shin HJ, Pack IS, Park JH, Kim HB, Kim CG. Metabolomic changes in grains of well-watered and drought-stressed transgenic rice. Journal of the Science of Food and Agriculture. 2016;**96**:807-814

[95] Zhang JY, Cruz-De-Carvaho MH, Torres-Jerez IV, Kang YU, Allen SN, Huhman DV, et al. Global reprogramming of transcription and metabolism in Medicavalhogotruncatula during progressive drought and after rewatering. Plant, Cell & Environment. 2014;**37**: 2553-2576

[96] Barchet GL, Dauwe R, Guy RD, Schroeder WR, Soolanayakanahally RY, Campbell MM, et al. Investigating the drought-stress response of hybrid poplar genotypes by metabolite profiling. Tree Physiology. 2014;**34**:1203-1209

[97] Nakabayashi R, Mori T, Saito K. Alternation of flavonoid accumulation under drought stress in *Arabidopsis thaliana*. Plant Signaling & Behavior. 2014;**9**:e29518

[98] Shelden MC, Dias DA, Jayasinghe NS, Bacic A, Roessner U. Root spatial metabolite profiling of two genotypes of barley (*Hordeum vulgare* L.) reveals differences in response to short-term salt stress. Journal of Experimental Botany. 1996;**67**(12):3731-3745. erw059

[99] Chen Y, Hoehenwarter W. Changes in the phosphoproteome and metabolome link early signaling events to rearrangement of photosynthesis and central metabolism in salinity and oxidative stress response in Arabidopsis. Plant Physiology. 2015;**169**(4):3021-3033. 01486

[100] Nam MH, Bang E, Kwon TY, Kim Y, Kim EH, Cho K, et al. Metabolite profiling of diverse rice germplasm and identification of conserved metabolic markers of rice roots in response to long-term mild salinity stress. International Journal of Molecular Sciences. 2015; **16**:21959-21974

[101] Meulebroek LV, Hanssens J, Steppe K, Vanhaecke L. Metabolic fingerprinting to assess the impact of salinity on carotenoid content in developing tomato fruits. International Journal of Molecular Sciences. 2016;**17**:821

[102] Cao D, Lutz A, Hill CB, Callahan DL, Roessner U. A quantitative profiling method of phytohormones and other metabolites applied to barley roots subjected to salinity stress. Frontiers in Plant Science. 2017;**7**

[103] Behr JH, Bouchereau A, Berardocco S, Seal CE, Flowers TJ, Zörb C. Metabolic and physiological adjustment of Suaeda maritima to combined salinity and hypoxia. Annals of Botany. 2017;**119**:965-976

[104] Lee SJ, Jeong EM, Ki AY, Oh KS, Kwon J, Jeong JH, et al. Oxidative defense metabolites induced by salinity stress in roots of *Salicornia herbacea*. Journal of Plant Physiology. 2016; **206**:133-142

[105] Zarza X, Atanasov KE, Marco F, Arbona V, Carrasco P, Kopka J, et al. Polyamine oxidase 5 loss-of-function mutations in *Arabidopsis thaliana* trigger metabolic and transcriptional reprogramming and promote salt stress tolerance. Plant, Cell & Environment. 2016;**40**: 527-542

[106] Mao G, Seebeck T, Schrenker D, Yu O. CYP709B3, a cytochrome P450 monooxygenase gene involved in salt tolerance in *Arabidopsis thaliana*. BMC Plant Biology. 2013;**13**:169

[107] Kiani-Pouya A, Roessner U, Jayasinghe NS, Lutz A, Rupasinghe T, Bazihizina N, et al. Epidermal bladder cells confer salinity stress tolerance in the halophyte quinoa and Atriplex species. Plant, Cell & Environment. 2017;**40**:1900-1915

[108] Bonhomme L, Benoît V, Tardieu F, Zivy M. Phosphoproteome dynamics upon changes in plant water status reveal early events associated with rapid growth adjustment in maize leaves. Molecular & Cellular Proteomics. 2012;**11**:957-972

[109] Hu Y, Guo S, Li X, Ren X. Comparative analysis of salt-responsive phosphoproteins in maize leaves using Ti^{4+}–IMAC enrichment and ESI-Q-TOF MS. Electrophoresis. 2013;**34**: 485-492

[110] Kim MH, Sonoda Y, Sasaki K, Kaminaka H, Imai R. Interactome analysis reveals versatile functions of *Arabidopsis*COLD SHOCK DOMAIN PROTEIN 3 in RNA processing within the nucleus and cytoplasm. Cell Stress & Chaperones. 2013;**18**:517-525

[111] Vialaret J, Di Pietro M, Hem S, Maurel C, Rossignol M, Santoni V. Phosphorylation dynamics of membrane proteins from Arabidopsis roots submitted to salt stress. Proteomics. 2014;**14**:1058-1070

[112] Mustafa G, Komatsu S. Quantitative proteomics reveals the effect of protein glycosylation in soybean root under flooding stress. Frontiers in Plant Science. 2014;**5**:627

[113] Picotti P, Aebersold R. Selected reaction monitoring-based proteomics: Workflows, potential, pitfalls and future directions. Nature Methods. 2012;**9**:555-566

[114] Picotti P, Clement-Ziza M, Lam H, Campbell DS, Schmidt A, Deutsch EW, et al. A complete mass-spectrometric map of the yeast proteome applied to quantitative trait analysis. Nature. 2013;**494**:266-270

[115] Khan MN, Sakata K, Hiraga S, Komatsu S. Quantitative proteomics reveals that peroxidases play key roles in post-flooding recovery in soybean roots. Journal of Proteome Research. 2014;**13**:5812-5828

[116] Ali GM, Komatsu S. Proteomic analysis of rice leaf sheath during drought stress. Journal of Proteome Research. 2006;**5**:396-403

[117] Cramer GR, Sluyter SCV, Hopper DW, Pascovici D, Keighley T, Haynes PA. Proteomic analysis indicates massive changes in metabolism prior to the inhibition of growth and photosynthesis of grapevine (*Vitis vinifera* L.) in response to water deficit. BMC Plant Biology. 2013;**13**:49

[118] Zhao F, Zhang D, Zhao Y, Wang W, Yang H, Tai F, et al. The difference of physiological and proteomic changes in maize leaves adaptation to drought, heat, and combined both stresses. Frontiers in Plant Science. 2016;**7**:1471

[119] Chen S, Gollop N, Heuer B. Proteomic analysis of salt-stressed tomato (*Solanum lycopersicum*) seedlings: Effect of genotype and exogenous application of glycinebetaine. Journal of Experimental Botany. 2009;**60**:2005-2019

[120] El Rabey HA, Al-Malki AL, Abulnaja KO. Proteome analysis of date palm (*Phoenix dactylifera* L.) under severe drought and salt stress. International Journal of Genomics. 2016;**7840759**:8

[121] Kamal AHM, Kim KH, Shin KH, Choi JS, Baik BK, et al. Abiotic stress responsive proteins of wheat grain determined using proteomics technique. AJCS. 2010;**4**:196-208

[122] Jiang F, Shen Y, Ma C, Zhang X, Cao W, Rui Y. Effects of TiO_2 nanoparticles on wheat (*Triticum aestivum L.*) seedlings cultivated under super-elevated and normal CO_2 conditions. PLoS One. 2017;**12**(5). DOI: 10.1371/journal.pone.0178088

Genetic Improvement of Tropical and Subtropical Fruit Trees via Biolistic Methods

Mousa Mousavi and Mohsen Brajeh Fard

Additional information is available at the end of the chapter

http://dx.doi.org/10.5772/intechopen.81373

Abstract

Biolistic is a special high-performance method for direct delivery of foreign DNA, RNA, or protein into plant cells. This method has less physiological risk on plant cell since there is no need for microbial intermediaries (*Agrobacterium* strains) and requires less additional DNA. Moreover, it can adapt for both monocotyledon and dicotyledonous plants. Recently, this method has also been successfully used to plant genome editing. Therefore, in this chapter, we discuss the application of this method for genetic improvement of some commercially important of tropical and subtropical fruit trees including banana, date palm, citrus, mango, olive, and pineapple. Also, we explain the details of biolistic protocols used for transient and stable gene expression in these fruit trees.

Keywords: gene gun, gene delivery, microprojectile bombardment, tropical fruits

1. Introduction

In the recent years, the scientists believe that the molecular methods have high potential for making gene delivery or genome editing possible in different plant species without altering their phenotypes. This capability is particularly valuable for fruit trees that have lengthy generation time and high levels of heterozygosity. In fact, the biotechnology methods now became as routine tools in biology research and plant transformation. So various methods had been introduced by the scientist for gene delivery to the plant cells (which may not be achievable by the traditional breeding methods), and subsequently they successfully regenerated without serious limitations [1–4]. Gene transferring to plant tissues can be achieved by two means: direct or indirect methods. In the direct methods, there is no need to *Agrobacterium* mediate, but the plasmids that are harboring desired DNA materials will deliver to the plant cells via physical or chemical means [5]. However, indirect gene transformation to plant tissues is usually achieved by mediated *Agrobacterium* strains. At the present time, in the most laboratories, gene delivery to plant tissues is achieved by mainly two means including biolistic and *Agrobacterium* methods [2, 4]. However, most of the gene transformation studies on fruit trees have been mediated by *Agrobacterium* strains, and biolistic has been less frequently used [6]. Infection with *Agrobacterium* may potentially produce unpredictable effects on the plant cells when transformed with T-DNA [7, 8]. The biolistic is a more applicable method for gene transformation in a wide range of plant cells and tissues [9], even those that could not transform by other transformation methods. In this method the precipitated DNA on gold or tungsten particles is transferred directly into the plant cells and tissues. Therefore, it is possible to introduce new traits with lower risk of the GMO effect with high reproducibility and no significant damage or artifacts [8]. Further, this method can be more adapted for breeding of plant species with a high degree of heterozygosity [10].

The biolistic method was introduced for the first time by Sanford [11]. Optimization of the transformation condition is very critical for achievement of an efficient protocol with high transformation frequency [12]. This strongly depends on the construct and promoter type and optimization of the physical and biological parameters. In order to achieve the best results with the biolistic method, the following are needed:

1. Appropriate construct (the type of genes and promoter)
2. Proper tissue (eases to regeneration as well as pretreatment prior to bombardment)
3. Optimized bombardment condition (biological parameters, as well as physical parameters, should been optimized)
4. Detecting of the insertion (integrated to the genome)

The biolistic method has a potential use for breeding of several tropical and subtropical fruit trees so that different genes were transferred to these trees for different purposes. Most of these genes are selectable and scorable marker genes which were used for the establishment of the optimized transformation protocols and some other genes of interest (which are encoding the economical traits).

One of the more permissible applications of the biolistic method is using it for genome editing or CRISPR in plants [13].

In this chapter, we explain the different gene transformation procedures introduced by scientists for various economically important tropical and subtropical fruit trees by the use of the biolistic method.

2. Banana

Several limitations had been reported for the breeding of banana cultivars through traditional methods mainly including long regenerating time, polyploidy, and male sterility [14, 15]. The biolistic method was successfully used for banana transformation so that several genes were transferred to different banana tissues for different purposes. However, this method may be integrated with the *Agrobacterium* to increase the efficiency of the gene transformation.

Embryogenic cells initiated from different tissues including immature male flowers [16], immature embryos [17], male inflorescence, and buds [18] were reported with high potential to gene transformation in banana and plantain. A protocol optimized for transient and stable transformation of the *uid*A gene in banana cells using a special gene gun is illustrated by [14]. The tungsten particles coated with various plasmids harboring *uid*A gene including pEmuGN (with Emu promoter), pBI-364, pBI-426, pBI-505 (with 35S promoter), and pAHC27 (with Ubi promoter) were delivered into banana cells and then comprised among them based on the level of transient expression after assayed with X-Gluc and MUG. The highest transient transformation was obtained with the pAHC27 plasmid. Also, the stable transformation was achieved after the bombardment of banana cells with pWRG1515 plasmid harboring *uid*A gene along with *hph* as a selectable marker gene (conferring resistance to hygromycin) and cultured on the medium contain 50 mg/L hygromycin.

Stable transformation of the Cavendish banana (*Musa* spp. AAA group) cv. Grand Nain was also reported by [16], using *uid*A and potential virus-resistance (BBTV) genes along with *npt*II gene as selectable marker gene using various plasmids (**Table 1**).

In other experiment [18], researchers transferred to the *Musa* spp. (AAB group) cv. Maçã the three plasmid constructions harboring *uid*A gene including pBI426 (70S promoter), pFF19 (70S promoter), and pCAMBIA1303 (35S promoter). The plasmids had been precipitated on the tungsten particles using 20 μL of spermidine and 50 μL of $CaCl_2$ and then accelerated to penetrate callus tissue located at 9 cm from stopping screen using 1100 psi helium pressure force. The transient expression was observed for all constructs, but the best result was obtained for pBI426 due to achievement of the highest regenerated plant after 3 months.

For obtaining a successful transformation through the biolistic method, it is important to reduce physical stress entered on target tissues promoted by bombardment shock waves. Bombarded tissues may reduce their regeneration potential especially in the case of embryogenic callus and immature tissues. Therefore, such sensitive tissues should bombard with lower helium pressures and target distance. In most studies on gene transformation of banana by biolistic methods, it had been found that best results were obtained in 1100–1350 psi helium pressure and 6–9 cm target distance (**Table 1**).

Another strategy for increasing the transformation frequency in biolistic method is the integrating biolistic with *Agrobacterium*-mediated transformation especially with monocotyledons plants. It has been found that the infection of the Gongjiao (*Musa acuminata* L. AA group, cv. Mas) floral apices with *Agrobacterium tumefaciens* (AGL1 contains pCAS04) suspension for 30 min after bombardment thrice with pCAS04 plasmid coated on the 0.6 μm gold particles under 1300 psi helium pressure force was increased transformation frequency 1.6- and 3.3-fold higher than that of gene gun and *Agrobacterium* methods, respectively [15].

2.1. Plant-based vaccine

Hepatitis B virus (*HBV*) is a worldwide disease causing chronic and acute infections in the human liver. Therefore, needful to produce a vaccine for this disease is very important. On the other hand, production of vaccines required a high cost whereas may not be possible to secure the large segment of the population in the world. An attempt was made by [19], to transfer the *HBsAg* gene, coding hepatitis B surface antigen to banana cv. Williams to make

Plant name	Explant type	Plasmid (s)	Reporter gene(s)/ promoter (s)	Selectable gene (s)/ promoter (s)	Helium pressure	Particle size (μm)/ type	Target distance (cm)	Osmoticum	Transformation efficiency	Reference
Musa spp. (ABB group) Bluggoe	Embryogenic suspension cells	pBI364, pBI426, pBI505, pEmuGN, pAHC27, pWRG1515	*uid*A/35S, Emu, Ubi	Hygromycin (*hph*)	4.5 bar	Tungsten	4		30%	[14]
Musa spp. (AAB group) Maçã	Immature male flowers	pBI426, pFF19, pCAMBIA1303	*uid*-A/neo/70S; *uid*-A/70S; *uid*-A/35S	Hygromycin	1100 psi	Tungsten	9		Best result was obtained with *uid*-A/*neo*/*70S*	[18]
Musa spp. (AAB group) Grand Nain	Immature male flower	pBT6.3-Ubi-NPT, pUbi-BTintORF1, pUbi-BTutORF5, pUGR73, pDHkan	BBTV intO1/Ubi pro, BBTV utO5/ Ubi pro, *uid*A/*Ubi* pro	*npt*II/BT6.3 pro, *npt* II/ CaMV 35S pro	550 KPa	1.0/gold	7.5		11%	[16]
Musa acuminata cv. Mas (AA)	Immature male flower	pCAMBIA-1301	*gus*/CaMV 35S	—	1100–1350 psi	1.0/gold	6		—	[17]
Musa acuminata L. (AA group, cv. Mas) Gongjiao	Floral apices	pCAS04	*uid*A, *npt*II/Ubi pro, actin pro	—	1300 psi	0.6/gold	4		9.8%	[15]
Musa sapientum cv. Rastali (AAA)	Bud	pBI333-EN4-RCC2, pMRC1301, pROKLa-Eg, pGEM.Ubi1-sgfps65T (GFP)	*npt*II/nopaline synthase gene, *gus*A and chitinase/rice actin 1, *npt*II/nopaline synthase gene (*nos*) promoter, soybean β-1,3-endoglucanse/ CaMV 35S, *gfp*/maize polyubiquitin 1 (Ubi1)		1100 psi		9		4–7.5%	[20]

Plant name	Explant type	Plasmid (s)	Reporter gene(s)/ promoter (s)	Selectable gene (s)/ promoter (s)	Helium pressure	Particle size (μm)/ type	Target distance (cm)	Osmoticum	Transformation efficiency	Reference
Citrus reticulata Blanco × *Citrus paradisi* Macf. cultivar Page	Embryogenic cells from suspension cultures		*gus*	*npt*II		Tungsten		0.3 M sorbitol + 0.3 M mannitol		[26]
Carrizo citrange (*Citrus sinensis* (L.) Osbeck × *Poncirus Trifoliate (L.) Raf.*), sweet orange (*Citrus sinensis* (L.) Osbeck) cv. Pera	Thin epicotyl sections	pE2113-GUS	*uid*A/CaMV 35S	*npt*II/NOS promoter	1550 psi	Tungsten M-25 (1.7)	6	0.2 M sorbitol + 0.2 M mannitol		[24]
Citrus macrophylla (C-mac)	Second and third newest leaves	CTV CP-CP interacting BiFC plasmids	*gfp*/35S	—	260–280 psi	0.6/gold	—	—		[8]
Olea europapea L. cv Canino	Somatic embryogenesis	pZ085 and pCGUδ0	*gus*/Ubi (sunflower)		580 kPa	Tungsten or gold				[44]
Olea europapea cv. "Picual"	Embryogenic callus	pCGUΔ1	*gus*/Ubi (sunflower)	*npt*II	900 psi	1.0/gold	6	0.2 mannitol	72.7%	[41]
Ananas comosus "Phuket" and "Pattavia"	Leaves of micropropagated shoots	AHC25	*gus*/maize Ubi	*bar*/maize ubiquitin promoter	1350 psi	Gold	7	0.2 M mannitol	66.7–86.4%	[29]
Ananas comosus L. cv. "Smooth Cayenne"	Callus	pDH-kan^R, pBS420, pART7.35S. GUS, pBS247. SCSV4.GUS, pGEM-Ubi-GFP	*gus*/35S or SCSV4, *gfp*/maize Ubi-1 and *ppo* gene (isolated from pineapple, for control of blackheart) under the control of 35S or maize Ubi-1	*npt*II/35S or SCSV4	1000 kPa	1.0/gold	18	—	0.21–1.5%	[32]

Plant name	Explant type	Plasmid (s)	Reporter gene(s)/ promoter (s)	Selectable gene (s)/ promoter (s)	Helium pressure	Particle size (μm)/ type	Target distance (cm)	Osmoticum	Transformation efficiency	Reference
Mangifera indica "Carabao" and "Kensington Pride"	Nucellar proembryonic masses	pBI426, pBINgfp-Ser	*gus*, *gfp* /CaMV 35S	*npt*II/*CaMV* 35S	125 psi	7/tungsten	15	0.2 M mannitol	1101 foci per microgram of DNA	[46]
Phoenix dactylifera L. "Estamaran"	Emberyogenic callus	pAct1-D	*gus*/5′ region of the rice actin 1		1100 psi	1.6/gold	9	0.4 M mannitol	1383 GUS blue spots/ bombardment	[39]
Phoenix dactylifera L. "Estamaran"	Somatic embryos	pAct1-D	*gus*/5′ region of the rice actin 1		1350 psi	0.6/gold	6	0.4 M mannitol	6–12 blue spots/ bombardment	[39]
Phoenix dactylifera L. "Siwy"	Emberyogenic callus	pBC4	Cholesterol oxidase gene/35S, *gus*/35S	Kan resistance/35S	1300 psi	Tungsten	9	0.2 M mannitol		[40]

Table 1. Description of gene transformation to some economically important tropical and subtropical fruit trees through biolistic method.

an alternative plant-based oral vaccine. After the bombardment of the banana meristems with pBHsAg plasmid vector harboring *bar* gene (inactivates phosphinothricin) as a selectable marker and *HBsAg* gene, they had detected the expression of antigen in banana which may have a potential to use it for security against this disease.

2.2. Disease resistance

Fusarium wilt race 1 is one of the limitation factors in banana production, caused by *Fusarium oxysporum* cubense f. sp. Due to cell wall of these fungi mainly made from chitin and β-1, 3-glucan, therefore, presence of chitinase and β-1,3-glucanase in banana tissues can increase the level of resistance to this disease. This was achieved by banana gene transformation with chitinase and β-1,3-glucanase genes using biolistic method [20]. They also transferred reporter genes *gfp* and *uid*A along with the chitinase and β-1,3-glucanase genes to detection of the transformation occurrence and subsequent expression in buds of Rastali cultivar (*Musa* spp. AAB group).

Black Leaf Streak Disease (BLSD) is another worldwide banana disease caused by *Mycosphaerella fijiensis*. The fungi induce streaks on the banana leaves which may lead to reduced fertility and may destroy the whole trees. On the other hand, infested plants usually produce a high level of free radicals, causing more challenges. In a research with goal to increase the level of banana tolerance to the BLSD reported by [21], they transferred two genes, including endochitinase (*ThEn-42*) and grape stilbene synthase (*StSy*) antifungal genes (with synergistic effect) together with chloroplastic (*chl*) Cu, Zn superoxide dismutase gene (*Cu, Zu-SOD*) (scavenging of free radical) to embryogenic callus of Cavendish banana (*Musa* spp. AAA group) cv. Grand Nain. After 4 years, the infection of the transgenic banana with these three genes was significantly reduced without any decrease in yield.

3. Citrus

The citrus breeding by traditional methods has some limitations including lengthy period of juvenility (8–10 years), polyembryony, incompatibility, parthenocarpy [22, 23], and high heterozygosity [24]. Molecular methods and gene transformation could be an alternative for breeding of the citruses and rapid regeneration with less time consumption. Currently, gene delivery into the epicotyl segments by *Agrobacterium*-mediated transformation is the most widely used method for gene transformation of the citruses. However, this approach has several drawbacks including the high number of chimeric or non-transformed plants due to the requirement for larger explant and gradient concentrations of the selective agent to the explant [24] and low regeneration frequency of stably transformed cells and recalcitrant of some citrus genotypes to *Agrobacterium* infection [23]. On the other hand, the biolistic method provides several advantages over *Agrobacterium*-mediated transformation such as high transformation efficiency, simplicity of the plasmid constructs which allows for the integration of larger inserts, the co-transformation of more than one construct, and less biological damage to the explant [23–25].

Evaluating the transient expression of a gene can provide valuable information in association with various properties of its produced protein, such as subcellular localization and intra–/intercellular trafficking, stability and degradation, expression levels, and interactions with other proteins [8]. In order to initiate a procedure for transient and stable transformation of the *uid*A/*npt*II genes to embryogenic cell suspension of citrus Tangelo (*Citrus reticulata* Blanco × *C. paradisi* Macf.) cultivar "Page," the researchers [26] used biolistic transformation method (**Table 1**).

Also, in other research [24], the *uid*A/*npt*II genes to thin epicotyl sections of the Carrizo citrange (*Citrus sinensis* (L.) Osbeck × *Poncirus trifoliata* (L.) Raf.) and sweet orange (*Citrus sinensis* (L.) Osbeck) cv. Pera were successfully delivered (**Table 1**). Recently the Carrizo immature epicotyl with another reporter gene *gfp* and also *npt*II gene as selectable marker through biolistic transformation are transferred [27].

Most reports on citrus gene transformation by biolistic were carried out on the transformation and expression detection of the selectable and scorable marker genes. However, result reported by [8] showed that the bombardment of the young leaves of the *Citrus macrophylla* (C-mac) with pSAT4-cEYFP-C1(B) harboring CPC^{TV}-GFP using Bio-Rad Helios gene-gun could have been causing the express of CP in the cytoplasm and nuclei of the epidermal cells.

4. Pineapple

The first report on the using of the biolistic method for gene transformation of pineapple was published by [28]. They introduced an efficient system for transformation of protocorm-like bodies with *gus*/*npt*II genes and then confirmed the gene insertions at one to three loci by Southern hybridization. After that, the published results [29–31] indicated that the pineapple cv. Phuket to herbicide Basta® X (with glufosinate ammonium as the active component) can be resisted by transforming with *bar* gene using biolistic transformation method. The transgenic plants showed herbicide tolerance when they were sprayed with herbicide (with twice the routine dose which used in the field) and remained green and healthy after 7 months, whereas the non-transformed plants became necrotic and died after 21 days. The stable integration of the *bar* gene in to the genome of the transformed plants was confirmed with PCR, RT-PCR, and Southern analyses after 380 days.

One of the physiological disorders which limited the industry of the pineapple in different area productions in the world such as Australia is the internal browning or blackheart. This disorder causes severe loss when appearing at conditions with day/night temperatures below 25/20°C with low light during fruit development and also during storage and shipment [32, 33]. To control the internal browning by the molecular breeding methods, an effort was made by [32] in order to obtain a transgene resistant to blackheart through biolistic method. The leaf callus of Smooth Cayenne cultivar was bombarded with gold particles coated with pART7 plasmid harboring PINPPO1 gene (pineapple polyphenol oxidase gene) which could successfully attain resistant plants to blackheart with an efficiency of 0.21–1.5% based on the PCR and Southern blot analysis (**Table 1**). Recent studies demonstrated that low temperature (5°C) could reduce blackheart through upregulated *AcGA2ox* gene and reduce GA_4 levels compared to the higher temperature (20°C) [33]. Also, the Del Monte Foods company introduces a red-fleshed pineapple "Rosé" by overexpression/suppression of some genes related to lycopene accumulation [34].

5. Date palm

One most important challenge face to genetical improvement of date palm through gene transformation and genome editing methods is difficult to regenerate in vitro due to lack of an efficient procedure for raped embryogenic callus induction. However, numerous successful protocols have been developed for regeneration of palm dates in in vitro conditions [35]. At present, shoot tips and immature inflorescence are mostly used for callus induction; however, several months and high levels of auxins (such as 2,4-D with100 mg/L concentration) are necessary that may induce epigenetic variation. Among the different tissues of date palm, the embryogenic callus and somatic embryos had more competencies to gene transformation [36]. Fortunately, the first report on date palm gene transformation had been done with biolistic method [37]. In this study embryogenic callus and somatic embryos of Kabkab cultivar were bombarded with gold particle coated with plasmid DNA construct carrying *gus* gene in different helium pressures (900, 1100, and 1350 psi) and target distances (6, 9, and 12 cm). The results indicated that highest *gus* expression in embryogenic callus was achieved when bombarded with 1100 psi/6 cm (helium pressures/target distance), whereas in somatic embryos, it was obtained in 1350 psi/9 cm. Date palm embryogenic callus exhibits the highest potential of transient expression (1383 *gus* blue spot per bombardment); however, somatic embryos present very lower potential of transient expression (9 ± 3 *gus* blue spot per bombardment). But they were more competent for attainment stable transformation [36, 38]. Unfortunately, the regeneration potential of embryogenic callus was dramatically decreased after bombardment due to shock wave. Recently, we introduce an efficient and optimized protocol for stable transformation of date palm Estamaran (Sayer) cultivar through biolistic transformation method [39]. Also, [40] developed a procedure for delivering the insecticidal cholesterol oxidase (*ChoA*) gene to embryogenic callus of Siwy cultivar through particle bombardment (**Table 1**). They transferred ChoA gene along with *gus* marker gene under control of 35S promoter and confirmed the insertions by *gus* assay, ELISA, and PCR.

6. Olive

Gene transformation to olive cultivars is considered as a difficult task due to recalcitrant nature of their tissues to regeneration process in vitro condition; however, it stays the most promising technique in respect to conventional and unconventional and even some biotechnological methods such as protoplast and somaclonal variation techniques. Classical methods of the olive breeding are more time-consuming, with very low efficient, due to lengthy seedling juvenile phase, alternation bearing, low fruitfulness, and low seed germinability [41–43].

The same as the other tropical fruit trees, the most of olive gene transformation studies were conducted using *Agrobacterium*-mediated transformation. However, there are few reports on the gene transformation by means of biolistic method in which most of them were down to optimization of scorable and selectable marker genes. Successfully transferred *gus* gene under the control of sunflower ubiquitin promoter in to small somatic embryos of Canino olive cultivar by biolistic method was reported by [44]. Afterward [45] bombarded the embryogenic tissues of Picual cultivar with three different plasmid constructs harboring *gus* gene under control of 35S, 35S with enhancer and sunflower ubiquitin promoters, and found that the ubiquitin promoter could significantly enhance the *gus* gene expression in olive.

More recently, [41] introduced an optimized protocol for transformation of olive cv. Picual embryogenic callus with *gus* gene under the control of sunflower ubiquitin promoter and *npt*II selective gene (**Table 1**) and achieved 72.7% transformation efficiency for embryogenic calli.

7. Mango

The result of [46] study reported an optimized protocol for transient and stable transformation of mango "Carabao" and "Kensington Pride" by biolistic method. They successfully optimized different bombardment parameters (**Table 1**), whereas more than thousand foci were observed per each nucellar proembryonic masses bombarded with a μg plasmid DNA. Afterwards [47], genetically transformed somatic embryos of the three mango varieties Haden, Madame Francis, and Kent with pCAMBIA 3201 construct harboring *gus* and *bar* genes by particle bombardment. After 3 months, only 4% embryos of Kent variety survived, while the other varieties did not survive. They confirmed integration of *gus* and *bar* genes by means of *gus* assay and PCR.

8. Conclusion

Gene transfer to tropical fruit trees via biolistic method can lower GMO risk. Therefore, it is recommended to use this method to gene transformation and particular genome editing via CRISPR technique. So plants can be genetically modified with low risk for humans and the environment.

Acknowledgements

The authors thank the IntechOpen Editorial Board for this publication and also would thank Mr. Muhammad Sarwar Khan for the invitation to write this chapter. There was no financial support for this study.

Conflict of interest

The authors declare that they have no conflict of interest.

Author details

Mousa Mousavi[1]* and Mohsen Brajeh Fard[2]

*Address all correspondence to: m.mousavi@scu.ac.ir

1 Department of Horticulture Science, Faculty of Agriculture, Shahid Chamran University of Ahvaz, Ahvaz, Iran

2 Department of Agronomy and Plant Breeding, Faculty of Agriculture, Shahid Chamran University of Ahvaz, Ahvaz, Iran

References

[1] Krishna H, Singh SK. Biotechnological advances in mango (*Mangifera indica* L.) and their future implication in crop improvement—A review. Biotechnology Advances. 2007;**25**(3):223-243. DOI: 10.1016/j.biotechadv.2007.01.001

[2] Rashid AHA, Lateef DD. Novel techniques for gene delivery into plants and its applications for disease resistance in crops. American Journal of Plant Sciences. 2016;**7**:181-193. DOI: 10.4236/ajps.2016.71019

[3] Tanuja P, Kumar AL. Transgenic fruit crops—A review. International Journal of Current Microbiology and Applied Sciences. 2017;**6**(8):2030-2037. DOI: 10.20546/ijcmas.2017.608.241

[4] Keshavareddy G, Kumar ARV, Vemanna SR. Methods of plant transformation—A review. International Journal of Current Microbiology and Applied Sciences. 2018;**7**(7):2656-2668. DOI: 10.20546/ijcmas.2018.707.312

[5] Anami S, Njuguna E, Coussens G, Aesaert S, Van Lijsebettens M. Higher plant transformation: Principles and molecular tools. The International Journal of Developmental Biology. 2013;**57**:483-494. DOI: 10.1387/ijdb.130232mv

[6] Litz RE, Padilla G. Genetic transformation of fruit trees. In: Schnell R, Priyadarshan P, editors. Genomics of Tree Crops. New York, NY: Springer; 2012. DOI: 10.1007/978-1-4614-0920-5_5

[7] Lacroix B, Vaidya M, Tzfira T, Citovsky V. The VirE3 protein of *Agrobacterium* mimics a host cell function required for plant genetic transformation. The EMBO Journal. 2005;**24**(2):428-437. DOI: 10.1038/sj.emboj.7600524

[8] Levy A, El-Mochtar C, Wang C, Goodin M, Orbovic V. A new toolset for protein expression and subcellular localization studies in citrus and its application to citrus tristeza virus proteins. Plant Methods. 2018;**14**:2. DOI: 10.1186/s13007-017-0270-7

[9] Bhatnagar S, Kapur A, Khurana P. Evaluation of parameters for high efficiency gene transfer via particle bombardment in Indian mulberry. Indian Journal of Experimental Biology. 2002;**40**:1387-1392

[10] Gardner RC. Gene transfer into tropical and subtropical crops. Scientia Horticulturae. 1993;**55**:65-82. DOI: 10.1016/0304-4238 (93)90025-L

[11] Sanford JC. The biolistic process. Trends in Biotechnology. 1988;**6**:299-302. DOI: 10.1016/0167-7799

[12] Klein TM. Particle bombardment: An established weapon in the arsenal of plant biotechnologists. In: Stewart N Jr, Touraev A, Citovsky V, Tzfira T, editors. Plant Transformation Technologies. Oxford: Wiley-Blackwell; 2011. DOI: 10.1002/9780470958988.ch3

[13] Lee DW, Kim JK, Lee S, Choi S, Kim S, Hwang I. Arabidopsis nuclear-encoded plastid transit peptides contain multiple sequence subgroups with distinctive chloroplast-targeting sequence motifs. The Plant Cell. 2008;**20**:1603-1622. DOI: 10.1105/tpc.108.060541

[14] Sagi L, Panis B, Remy S, Schoofs H, De Smet K, Swennen R, et al. Genetic transformation of banana and plantain (*Musa* spp.) via particle bombardment. Nature Biotechnology. 1995;**13**(5):481. DOI: 10.1038/nbt0595-481

[15] Liu J, Gao P, Sun X, Zhang J, Sun P, Wang J, et al. Efficient regeneration and genetic transformation platform applicable to five *Musa* varieties. Electronic Journal of Biotechnology. 2017;**25**:33-38. DOI: 10.1016/j.ejbt.2016.11.002

[16] Becker DK, Dugdale B, Smith MK, Harding RM, Dale JL. Genetic transformation of Cavendish banana (*Musa* spp. AAA group) cv 'Grand Nain' via microprojectile bombardment. Plant Cell Reports. 2000;**19**(3):229-234. DOI: 10.1007/s002990050004

[17] Chee WW, Jalil M, Abdullah MO, Othman RY, Khalid N. Comparison of beta-glucuronidase expression and anatomical localization in bombarded immature embryos of banana cultivar mas via biolistic transformation. Asia-Pacific Journal of Molecular Biology and Biotechnology. 2005;**13**(1):15-22

[18] Houllou-Kido LM, Kido EA, Falco MC, Silva Filho MDC, Figueira AVDO, Nogueira NDL, et al. Somatic embryogenesis and the effect of particle bombardment on banana Maçã regeneration. Pesquisa Agropecuária Brasileira. 2005;**40**(11):1081-1086. DOI: 10.1590/S0100-204X2005001100005

[19] Elkholy SF, Ismail RM, Bahieldin A, Sadik AS, Madkour MA. Expression of hepatitis B surface antigen (HBsAg) gene in transgenic banana (*Musa* Spp.). Arab Journal of Biotechnology. 2009;**12**:291-302. DOI: 10.4172/0974-276X-C1-104

[20] Subramaniam S, Mahmood M, Meon S, Rathinam X. Genetic engineering for tolerance to *Fusarium* wilt race 1 in *Musa sapientum* cv. Rastali (AAB) using biolistic gun transformation system. Tree and Forestry Science and Biotechnology. 2010;**4**(2):65-75

[21] Vishnevetsky J, White TL, Palmateer AJ, Flaishman M, Cohen Y, Elad Y, et al. Improved tolerance toward fungal diseases in transgenic Cavendish banana (*Musa* spp. AAA group) cv. Grand Nain. Transgenic Research. 2011;**20**(1):61-72. DOI: 10.1007/s11248-010-93927

[22] Moore GA, Rogers KL, Kamps TL, Pajon M, Stover J, Febres VJ, et al. Rapid cycling plant breeding in citrus. In: Metarex® 4% Snail and Slug Bait. 2016. p. 80

[23] Febres V, Fisher L, Khalaf A, Moore GA. Citrus transformation: Challenges and prospects. In: Genetic Transformation. Rijeka: InTech; 2011

[24] Bespalhok Filho JC, Kobayashi AK, Pereira LF, Galvão RM, Vieira LG. Transient gene expression of beta-glucuronidase in citrus thin epicotyl transversal sections using particle bombardment. Brazilian Archives of Biology and Technology. 2003;**46**(1):1-6. DOI: 10.1590/S1516-89132003000100001

[25] Dönmez D, Şimşek Ö, Kaçar YA. Genetic engineering techniques in fruit science. International Journal of Environmental & Agriculture Research (IJOEAR). 2016;**2**(12): 115-128

[26] Yao JL, Wu JH, Gleave AP, Morris BA. Transformation of citrus embryogenic cells using particle bombardment and production of transgenic embryos. Plant Science. 1996;**113**(2):175-183. DOI: 10.1016/0168-9452(95)04292-X

[27] Wu H, Acanda Y, Jia H, Wang N, Zale J. Biolistic transformation of Carrizo citrange (*Citrus sinensis* Osb. × *Poncirus trifoliata* L. Raf.). Plant Cell Reports. 2016;**35**(9):1955-1962. DOI: 10.1007/s00299-016-2010-2

[28] Nan GL, Nagai C. Genetic transformation of pineapple (*Ananas comosus* [L.] Merr.) via particle bombardment. In Vitro Cellular and Developmental Biology Animal. 1998;**34**:1052

[29] Sripaoraya S, Marchant R, Power JB, Davey MR. Herbicide-tolerant transgenic pineapple (*Ananas comosus*) produced by microprojectile bombardment. Annals of Botany. 2001;**88**(4):597-603. DOI: 10.1006/anbo.2001.150

[30] Sripaoraya S, Keawsompong S, Insupa P, Davey MR, Power JB, Srinives P. Evaluation of transgene stability, gene expression and herbicide tolerance of genetically modified pineapple under field conditions. Acta Horticulturae. 2006;(702):37-40. DOI: 10.17660/ActaHortic.2006.702.3

[31] Sripaoraya S, Keawsompong S, Insupa P, Davey MR, Power JB, Srinives P. Genetically manipulated pineapple: Transgene stability, gene expression and herbicide tolerance under field conditions. Plant Breeding. 2006;**125**:411-413. DOI: 10.1111/j.1439-0523.2006.01229.x

[32] Ko HL, Campbell PR, Jobin-Décor MP, Eccleston KL, Graham MW, Smith MK. The introduction of transgenes to control blackheart in pineapple (*Ananas comosus* L.) cv. Smooth Cayenne by microprojectile bombardment. Euphytica. 2006;**150**(3):387. DOI: 10.1007/s10681-006-9124-5

[33] Zhang Q, Rao X, Zhang L, He C, Yang F, Zhu S. Mechanism of internal browning of pineapple: The role of gibberellins catabolism gene (AcGA2ox) and GAs. Scientific Reports. 2016;**6**:33344. DOI: 10.1038/srep33344

[34] Ogata T, Yamanaka S, Shoda M, Urasaki N, Yamamoto T. Current status of tropical fruit breeding and genetics for three tropical fruit species cultivated in Japan: Pineapple, mango, and papaya. Breeding Science. 2016;**66**(1):69-81. DOI: 10.1270/jsbbs.66.69

[35] Al-Khayri JM, Jain SM, Johnson DV. Date Palm Biotechnology Protocols, Volume 1: Tissue Culture Applications, Methods in Molecular Biology. New York: Humana Press; 2017. 1637p. DOI: 10.1007/978-1-4939-7156-5

[36] Mousavi M, Mousavi A, Habashi A, Arzani K. Optimization of physical and biological parameters for transient expression of *uid*A gene in embryogenic callus of date palm (*Phoenix dactylifera* L.) via particle bombardment. African Journal of Biotechnology. 2009;**8**:3721-3730

[37] Mousavi M, Mousavi A, Habashi AA, Arzani K. Investigation on ability of date palm gene transformation. In: Proceedings of 5th Iranian Horticultural Sciences Congress. Iran: Shiraz University; 2007. p. 244

[38] Mousavi M, Mousavi A, Habashi AA, Arzani K, Dehsara B. Transient transformation of date palm via *Agrobacterium*-mediated and particle bombardment. Emirates Journal of Food and Agriculture. 2014;**26**(6):528-539. DOI: 10.9755/ejfa.v26i6.16754

[39] Mousavi M, Mousavi A, Habashi AA, Arzani K, Dehsara B, Brajeh M. Genetic transformation of date palm via microprojectile bombardment. In: Al-Khayri J, Jain S, Johnson D, editors. Date Palm Biotechnology Protocols Volume I. New York, NY: Humana Press; 2017. pp. 269-280. DOI: 10.1007/978-1-4939-7156-5_22

[40] Allam MA, Saker MM. Microprojectile bombardment transformation of date palm using the insecticidal cholesterol oxidase (ChoA) gene. In: Date Palm Biotechnology Protocols Volume I. New York, NY: Humana Press; 2017. pp. 281-293. DOI: 10.1007/978-1-4939-7156-5_23

[41] Pérez-Barranco G, Torrebl Lavianca R, Padilla IM, Sánchez-Romero C, Pliego-Alfaro F, Mercado JA. Studies on genetic transformation of olive (*Olea europaea* L.) somatic embryos: I. Evaluation of different aminoglycoside antibiotics for nptII selection; II. Transient transformation via particle bombardment. Plant Cell, Tissue and Organ Culture (PCTOC). 2009;**97**(3):243-251. DOI: 10.1007/s11240-009-9520-3

[42] Rugini E, Gutiérrez Pesce P. Genetic improvement of olive. Pomologia Croatica. 2006; **12**(1):43-74. DOI: 10.1016/j.biotechadv.2016.03.004

[43] Rugini E, Cristofori V, Silvestri C. Genetic improvement of olive (*Olea europaea* L.) by conventional and in vitro biotechnology methods. Biotechnology Advances. 2016;**34**(5): 687-696. DOI: 10.1016/j.biotechadv.2016.03.004

[44] Lambardi M, Benelli C, Amorosi S, Branca C, Caricato G, Rugini E. Microprojectile-DNA delivery in somatic embryos of olive (*Olea europaea* L.). In: III International Symposium on Olive Growing. 1997. pp. 505-510

[45] Pliego-Alfaro F, Pérez-Barranco G, Sánchez-Romero C, Mercado JA. Genetic transformation of olive somatic embryos through biolistic. In: International Symposium

on Biotechnology of Temperate Fruit Crops and Tropical Species; 10-14 October, 2005. Florida USA: Hilton Daytona Beach/Ocean Walk Village Daytona Beach; 2005. p. 166

[46] Cruz-Hernande A, Town L, Cavallaro A, Botella JR. Transient and stable transformation in mango by particle bombardment. Acta Horticulturae. 2000;**509**:237-242

[47] Chavarri M, Vegas A, Za mbrano AY, Demey JR. Transformación de embriones somáticos de mango por biobalística. Interciencia. 2004;**29**(5):261-266

Chapter 7

Molecular Approaches to Address Intended and Unintended Effects and Substantial Equivalence of Genetically Modified Crops

Lerato B.T. Matsaunyane and Ian A. Dubery

Additional information is available at the end of the chapter

http://dx.doi.org/10.5772/intechopen.80339

Abstract

The release of GM organisms into the environment and marketing of GM crops have resulted in public debate in many parts of the world. This debate is likely to continue, probably in the broader context of plant biotechnology and consequences for human societies. The general issues under debate include cost–benefit analysis and safety issues, but might exhibit regional differences and crop-specific nuances. This chapter addresses an in-depth understanding of events involved in transgene insertion, but also the unintended effects of transformation following the production of genetically enhanced plants. In order to dissect this topic, a foundational overview is given on biolistic- and Agrobacterium-based techniques. Background information of possible transformation-induced unintended alterations to transgenic plant genomes is reviewed and aspects that collectively constitute possible unintended transformation - and post-transformation events are described. This is followed by an overview of molecular techniques to study gene insertion and – expression with special focus on differential gene expression analysis techniques to investigate unintended effects of genetic transformation. Historical and current safety assessment guidelines and requirements are also briefly discussed.

Keywords: intended effects, molecular analysis, transgenic plants, substantial equivalence, unintended effects

1. Introduction

The modern biotechnology era as applied to crop production was initiated by molecular marker-assisted selection to select agriculturally important traits [1]. Other developments included recombinant DNA technology which helped breeders by providing a diverse gene pool for trait selection, targeted deletion or insertions of genes into genomes, and site-directed mutagenesis to modify gene functions [2]. GM crops have been developed over the years for improvement of desired traits for enhanced agricultural production, as well as to facilitate reduced use of agricultural pesticides [3]. The technology employed to produce GM crops has been described as advantageous when compared to conventional plant breeding, since the desired traits can be obtained in a relatively shorter period of time. In addition, the technology may enable the introduction of desired characteristics that cannot be accomplished solely through conventional plant breeding.

In view of the global population increases, factors that have been considered important to cope with the increasing food demand include the development of crop varieties with improved nutrition and high yield in different climatic conditions, development of varieties that require the use of less water and fertilizers, and the production of varieties with enhanced resistance against abiotic and biotic stresses [4]. Moreover, new varieties should exhibit high storage quality and appropriate features for processing and market consumption. Specific traits that have been used to improve crops include herbicide - and insect resistance, salt and drought tolerance, increased yield, high protein content and vitamin A enrichment.

Pest-resistant and herbicide tolerant varieties were the first products of GM technologies and they were commercialized in the mid-1990s. In general, farmers have widely accepted GM technologies and the use of GM crops has expanded rapidly in developing countries [5]. The expected expiration of patents on earlier varieties of GM crops will serve as an opportunity for other companies to produce alternative varieties that may compete within the GMO market, thus challenging existing GM varieties. In addition, it will elicit innovative competition in terms of traits to be investigated which were previously not considered. It is therefore important to ensure that existing and future GM crops and - products created through recombinant DNA technology are assessed with regards to any potential risk they may have on human, animal and environmental health.

2. Benefits and limitations of genetically modified crops

One of the highlighted advantages of GM crops, among others, is their ability of these to enhance food security, particularly to small-scale and resource-poor farmers in developing countries [6]. Some of the noted benefits include increased crop yield in a relatively shorter period of time, reduction in the utilization and cost of plant protection chemicals, crops with enhanced tolerance to environmental stresses, reduction in labor input, and production of foods that are affordable with enhanced nutritional contents [6]. These benefits have been said to, overall, improve agricultural production and plant breeding in developing countries.

However, the documented benefits have been countered by shortcomings and concerns. Some of the issues brought forward include potential toxicity, the assumption that the products may contain allergens and the possible development of antibiotic resistance from the utilization of GM products [7]. Genetically, concerns about GM crops include the possible unintended transfer of genes from GM to non-GM crops or to their wild type relatives, the evolution of GM crops into becoming weeds, the direct and indirect impact of GM crops on non-target species, environmental risks associated with GM crops, and the impact of GM crops on genetic diversity [8]. Directed at the small-scale and resource-poor farmers, the highlighted concerns also include hindrances that may result in limited access to seeds created by patents on the GM crops [9]. Furthermore, contrary to the highlighted benefits of GM crops, crops with enhanced resistance have been viewed as having a one-sided benefit to commercial farmers that grow the crops and companies that own the production technologies [8, 10].

3. Transformation techniques used for the production GM crops

Transgenic technology deals with the integration of exogenous DNA into the plant genome using gene transfer technologies [11]. While newer methods such as nanoparticle-mediated delivery are in development, two methods are predominantly used for exogenous DNA transfer into plants; Agrobacterium-mediated transformation and particle bombardment. The first is an indirect or vector-based transformation method, and utilizes the ability of *Agrobacterium tumefaciens* bacteria to copy and transfer a specific portion of DNA (T-DNA) present on a tumor-inducing (Ti) plasmid into the nucleus of the plant cell. This allows for the integration of the DNA into chromosomes and subsequently leading to the integration of the T-DNA into the plant genome. This type of transformation involves three stages [12]. The initiation stage entails the insertion of the gene of interest into a suitable functional construct. The construct includes the gene expression promoter, gene of interest, selectable marker as well as codon modification. The initiation stage then continues to the insertion of the transgene into the Ti-plasmid. The final step of the initiation stage involves the insertion of the T-DNA, which contains the transgene, into Agrobacterium. The next stage is the bacterium-to-plant transfer during which the transformed bacteria are mixed with plant cells to facilitate the transfer of T-DNA into the plant genome. The final stage is nucleus targeting where the transgene is randomly integrated into the plant chromosome. Following nucleus targeting, non-homologous end-joining processes [13] enables the integration of T-DNA into the plant genome in the absence of any homology between the T-DNA and plant DNA sequences [14]. The possible need for tissue culture steps on selective artificial media associated with Agrobacterium transformation may lead to somoclonal variations, which in itself may lead to genetic changes in the host genome.

In contrast, biolistic transformation is commonly used to transform plants that are not susceptible to Agrobacterium transformation [15]. The integration of transgenes into a host plant genome, following particle bombardment, generally occurs non-randomly at AT-rich regions carrying nuclear matrix attachment region (MAR) motifs [16]. These elements have been postulated to be target sites for transgene integration into the host plant genome [16, 17]. Their function has been explained as creating open chromatin to make the host plant genome accessible to transgenes.

Both Agrobacterium and biolistic methods may be used for chloroplast/plastid transformation [18], but is applicable to only a relatively small number of crops. Chloroplast transformation is attractive because of its maternal inheritance, ensuring is a strong level of biological containment [18].

Newer techniques for genome editing include zinc finger nucleases (ZFNs), TAL effector nucleases (TALENs), and very importantly, the CRISPR/Cas9 (Clustered Regularly Interspaced Short Palindromic Repeats/CRISPR associated protein) system. The latter shows much promise for genetic modification and its versatility to modify the genome contributed to the current genome editing revolution [19].

Transformation methodology that include viral delivery systems is consistently being improved and recent advances in nanotechnology may overcome some of the limitations of the conventional methods in regards to species-independent passive delivery of transgenes [20].

4. Integration of transgenes into plant genomes: Aspects of possible unintended effects in transgenics

Single copy or repeated or multiple insertions of exogenous DNA may occur during genetic engineering transformation [21]. In addition, multiple insertions can take place into linked or unlinked sites [22, 23]. Moreover, following transformation, the transgene may be unstable within the host genome, and the insertion site may also be unstable owing to the transgene instability [24, 25].

Directed and inverted repeats are some of the complex integration patterns which have been found to result from Agrobacterium-mediated transformation [26]. Inversion [23] and translocations [27] have been found to be some of the types of chromosomal rearrangements linked to T-DNA insertion occurring at the insertion site in the plant genome. Vector-based filler DNA (non-T-DNA sequence from the transformation vector backbone) has also been observed following the integration of exogenous DNA into the plant genome. Plant-based filler DNA has been found between T-DNA repeats [25, 28], whereas vector-based filler DNA sequences were found outside the left and right borders of the T-DNA [29]. The plant-based filler DNA is regarded as an important facilitator of the integration of T-DNA into plant chromosomes [25].

Agrobacterium-based integration occasionally causes the recurrent integration of T-DNA vector backbone sequences into the transgenic plant genome [30]. It is possible to have vector backbone flanking the right border (RB) integrated into the host plant genome following transgene insertion [31]. This event has been hypothesized to be the result of T-DNA processing that occurred where, instead of the insertion initiated at from the RB, this initiation site is skipped and T-DNA insertion occurs from the LB.

Transformation methods directed at the chloroplast has the advantage of minimizing the insertion of unnecessary DNA that may accompany nuclear genome transformation. Furthermore, gene insertion into the chloroplast genome is not associated with inadvertent inactivation of a host gene due to transgene integration and, due to a less compact chromatin structure, does not exhibit positional effects [18].

5. Distribution of transgene integration sites

Predictions into the fate and integration site of a transgene into the plant genome are not possible, based on the genome's nucleotide sequence of the host genome [32]. Several authors have used various genetic mapping techniques to demonstrate that, in several plants species, transgenes integrate throughout the entire plant genome without any preference for a specific chromosome [33]. However, T-DNA containing transgenes have been found to show preference toward gene-rich regions [22, 34]. This preference has been found to be responsible for disruptions to endogenous gene functions.

Several cytological methods have been employed to detect transgene chromosomal location and structure, and these include genomic *in situ* hybridization (GISH) and fluorescence *in situ* hybridization (FISH) [35, 36]. These methods have assisted some researchers in identifying the transgene integration site/s at the sub-telomeric and telomeric regions of individual chromosomes [37].

In addition to the cytological methods, identification of the transgene insertion site has been done through direct sequencing of flanking DNA followed by the rescue of clones carrying transgene/genomic DNA junctions [24, 33, 38]. A high correlation was found between complex integration patterns and transgenic loci with unstable gene expression [23, 24, 39]. As a result, it was concluded that the determining factors of the stability of an expressed gene are the site as well as the structure of the integration site. In addition, it was found that the locus of transgene integration and the regions surrounding the insertion site are crucial for the stable expression of a transgene [15, 35].

Studies of transgenic tobacco indicated that chromosome telomeres are preferred by stable inserts where no binary vector sequence is present [35]. On the other hand, the integration of transgenes was found to have preference for the distal part of chromosome arms which are gene-rich regions [34, 40]. This preferred integration was found to be true in monocot species [37] and petunia [41].

During the integration of a transgene into the plant genome, a disruption may occur within the DNA and it is important to establish whether the disruption is contrary to an event that may occur during natural recombination mechanisms. Furthermore, the transgene site of integration must be clearly analyzed to investigate whether this site is not an active gene-rich region, thus causing changes to biochemical pathways within the plant. Sequence data of the regions flanking the transgene following the T-DNA insertion into the tobacco genome revealed the frequent presence of motifs, and include microsatellite sequences, AT-rich sequences characteristic of matrix-attached regions, retro-elements and tandem repeats [39]. MARs are important for the expression of integrated reporter genes, the protection of transgenes from position effects, serve as the replication origin, as well as targeting transgene integration into the host genome [13]. Several authors evaluated the junction regions in transgene loci and found genomic sequences that contained AT-rich MARs elements [13].

In contrast to the random insertion of the Agrobacterium – and biolistic methods targeted at the nuclear genome, chloroplast transformation involves homologous recombination with sequences flanking the insertion site and transgene integration is therefore more specific and predictable [18].

6. General views on the safety of GM crops

Some consumer concerns brought forward were regarding the safety of GM crops, food and feed [42]. As a result, the production of GM crops led to increased investigations within government regulatory boards in terms of research required to determine the safety of these products [43]. Activists, particularly in Europe, have intensified their opposition to the introduction and production of GM crops, food and feed [44]. To date, no international consensus has been reached for evaluation of the safety of GM plants for consumption. Over the last decade, the safety of GM crops has been routinely tested in some countries and protein- and DNA-based methods have been developed for testing of GM crops. Worldwide, legislation now faces questions on the use and labeling requirements of GM crops and their derivatives. However, there are still concerns about the safety of GM crops [9, 45]. Also, GM crops could contain toxic substances produced as by-products of the expression of the transgene. Moreover, the GM crops might not be substantially equivalent at the genome-, proteome- and metabolome levels to traditional untransformed counterparts due to possible disruption of the expression of endogenous genes.

Extensive safety assessments are an important component of the production of GM crops [46]. There are factors that are essential to interrogate to understand the impact of the expression of the "foreign" transgene on the expression of endogenous genes and on the host plant as a whole [32, 47].

7. Safety assessment of GM crops, food and feed

The current techniques utilized for the safety assessment of derivatives of genetically modified crops, particularly food- and feed-based derivatives, evolved from collaborations between international agencies, which include the United Nations' World Health Organization (WHO) and Food and Agricultural Organization [48] and the Organization for Economic Co-ordination and Development [49]. The techniques entail a comparative assessment between the characteristics of the modified crop and an existing crop, which is usually the parent crop from which the genetic modification was developed.

Research conducted by the International Council for Science (ICSU) and the FAO, showed no evidence of adverse effects of GM crops on the environment as well as no toxicity presented by the consumption of foods derived from GM crops [50, 51]. The results further showed that gene transfer that occurred from GM crops to the wild-type relative was similar to the occurrence obtained from traditional crops. Further research conducted on the environmental impact of GM crops found no evidence of negative effects [52].

Concerns that have been raised in terms of the safety of GM crops, environmental risks, protection of biodiversity and impact on human and animal health have been investigated through the Cartagena Protocol on Biosafety (Secretariat of the Convention on Biological Diversity 2000). This protocol has been used by countries to develop national GMO regulatory frameworks. Details required for application of the release of GMOs include a description of the GM plant, the GM trait, as well as the country of origin of the GM plant. Furthermore, requirements include general information on the release of the GM plant, description of GM-derived products and uses, and description of field trials undertaken for the GM plant. In addition, details required for the release of the GM plant include description of the pollen spreading characteristics of the GM plant, handling of seeds and the vegetative reproduction methods of the plant. Moreover, information is required on transgenes and their respective products, which include information such as transgene expression levels, declaration on whether the expression is constitutive or induced and expression site on the plant. Additionally, information on the potential resistance to environmental or biological conditions, potential risks to human and animal health, potential long-term impact of the GM plant on biotic and abiotic components of the environment, and socio-economic impact of the GM plant on communities in the proposed release region. The release also requires information on how the GM plant will be monitored, how possible pathogenic and ecologically disruptive impacts will be evaluated, how unused parts of the GM plant will be disposed of and measures that will be used for risk management [42].

8. Outcomes of safety assessment, substantial equivalence, intended and unintended effects

As defined by the European Commission, three possible outcomes exist following safety assessment studies. Firstly, the modified food can be similar to the traditional food or ingredient, thus eliminating the need for further testing. Secondly, the modified food can be homologous to the traditional food, with some distinctly characterized differences, in which case safety assessments targeted at the differences must be performed. Thirdly, the modified food can stand apart from the traditional counterpart in numerous and complicated aspects, or no traditional counterpart is available. In this instance, the modified food will require a comprehensive assessment similar to that discussed by König et al. [47]. This may be due to the fact that the endogenous genes and their functions will possibly be disrupted through the random integration of the transgene in the plant DNA. These effects of transformation are termed 'unintended' or 'non-target' effects as they occur secondary to the primary aim of crop improvement [46].

Prior to studying the possible unintended effects of recombinant DNA techniques, it is important to understand the definitions of these effects. There are intended effects of genetic engineering and these are changes that occur following genetic modifications which are aimed to take place as a result of the introduction of the transgene and will consequently result in the accomplishment of the original objective of the genetic engineering process [32]. Unintended effects are those changes that occur following genetic engineering where significant differences are found in the response, phenotype and composition of the GM plant when compared with the traditional plant from which it is derived.

Unintended effects have further been divided into 'predicable' and 'unpredictable' unintended effects [32]. Predictable unintended effects are changes that exceed the primary expected effects of the introduction of the transgene, but are, however, applicable through the aid of the current knowledge of plant biology and metabolic pathways. On the other hand, unpredictable unintended effects are changes that are currently undefined and not clearly understood. Methods that can be exploited to determine the presence of unintended outcomes of transformation include, among others, determining the transgene integration site/s, the events that occur during the integration of the transgene into the host plant, as well as gene expression analysis of the transgenic genome compared to the traditional counterpart, thus showing the impact of transformation on the expression of endogenous genes.

9. The need for molecular characterization of GM crops

Guidelines have been set for the molecular characterization of GM crops prior to market and commercial release and these were placed in six categories [53]. These categories are (i) description of the genetic material used for the transformation, including the origin of the donor organism and how the gene was isolated, (ii) description of the transformation method, (iii) description of the transgene loci, (iv) transcript and protein characterization, (v) inheritance and stability of the transgene and (vi) detection and identification of the transgene.

The specified requirements under (i) include information on the plasmid used in the production of the recombinant, detailing genetic elements such as the orientation and position of the transgene expression cassette within the vector, the restriction endonuclease sites of the transformation construct and clearly marked T-DNA borders and promoters. In order to comply, the number of insertion events of the transgene must also be supplied, as well as the transgene insertion site(s). Insertion site detection is expected to be presented as the transgene sequence accompanied by approximately 500 bp of plant DNA in both flanking regions. Possible novel chimeric open reading frames (ORF) should be described and their functionality evaluated. If the flanking sequence contains part of the chimeric ORF, it is expected that more sequencing must be performed beyond the 500 bp radius until a putative ORF is obtained.

Requirements regarding the expression of the transgene entail, among others, details on the translation of the transcript to protein, tissue specificity of the transcript and protein expression, as well as levels of expression. Furthermore, information on the biochemical, molecular and physiological properties of the transgene product is required as well as the stability of the protein(s) in the cell and in the surrounding environment.

It is quite evident that extensive molecular analyses are required for safety assessments, the main objective being the need to demonstrate that GM crops are equivalent to their traditional counterparts, (*i.e.* substantial equivalence), and that there are no introductions of any additional or new risks to consumer health [32]. These assessments are put in place to quantitatively detect or identify the GM crops, food and feed that are being introduced into the market [54].

10. Molecular comparison of transgenic plants: Genome and transcriptome approaches

Several molecular marker techniques that have successfully been used for various research applications, such as cultivar identification, identification of genes for important agricultural traits and marker-assisted selection, can also be applied toward transgenic crops [55]. Molecular marker technologies may therefore serve as rapid and cost-effective methods for genome comparison and as such may be used as an initial screen of recombinant plants.

Simple Sequence Repeats (SSRs), also known as microsatellites, are tandem short oligonucleotide repeat sequences flanked by conserved DNA sequences that can be used to obtain a DNA-based fingerprint of the plant under investigation and are reliable and efficient [56, 57]. Microsatellites are regarded as advantageous as they are simple to perform, low amounts of DNA are required, highly reproducible and the ability to detect high levels of polymorphism [56]. A related marker technique that has been introduced in transgenic crop research is retrotransposon-based markers. The novelty of this technique stems from its ability to reveal extensive chromosomal distribution, as well as randomized genome distribution [58, 59]. Random Amplified Polymorphic DNA (RAPD) techniques are suitable for studies focused on the identification of specific and desired traits and the identification of clonal variants [56], while mutations, insertions and deletions to specific chromosomes or chromosomal regions can be studied through the Restriction Fragment Length Polymorphism (RFLP) technique [60]. For the determination of the insertion site of a transgene and filler DNA, gene-walking methods from known into unknown sequences can be applied [61].

An older technique for gene expression analysis was Northern (mRNA) blotting that only allowed the analysis of a single gene per study. However, developments have facilitated analysis of differential gene expression, or transcript profiling, where the expression of a multitude of genes can be simultaneously analyzed. Differential gene expression has been divided into two categories, namely closed and open architecture systems [62]. A closed system is one where the genes of interest are known and the genome from which the genes are derived has been well characterized [62]. On the other hand, open systems are those that do not require prior knowledge of the transcriptome, as well as the genome of origin.

Several methods, alone or in combination, might be appropriate for optimal gene expression profiling in transgenic plants. Some examples include (not exclusively): Serial Analysis of Gene Expression (SAGE), a gene expression method which allows for quantification and analysis of genes with unknown sequences [63]. This method employs two processes which entail the production of short sequence tags (STTs) from cDNA followed by linking and cloning of these tags for sequencing. LongSAGE enables transcriptome analysis of increased lengths which in turn improves the accuracy of annotating genes [64].

Microarrays provide a global view of gene expression and are found in two forms; DNA-fragment-based and oligonucleotide-based microarrays [65] with the source of array fragments being either anonymous genomic clones, EST clones or ORF amplified DNA fragments. The advantage of this technique is that a range of both weak and strong signals can be monitored on the same microarray, enabling the simultaneous analysis of a large number of genes. In addition, the technique allows for a pair-wise comparison of samples [66]. However, a major disadvantage of this technique is that an accurate sequence database must be available to facilitate the construction of the microarrays, as well as a large amount of mRNA as starting material to perform the gene expression analysis [65].

With the advent of next-generation sequencing, RNA sequencing (RNASeq or whole transcriptome shotgun sequencing), was developed. RNA-Seq is used to analyze changes in the different RNA species comprising the cellular transcriptome and can inform on the presence and quantity of RNAs in plant samples [67]. Specifically, RNA-Seq facilitates the ability to look at genetic alterations, mutations and changes in gene expression, or differences in gene expression in different groups or treatments such as transgenic – *vs.* conventional plants.

However, all of the above techniques require substantial amount of sequence information of the genome under investigation. Moreover, availability of funding is another factor for consideration. As a result, alternative gene expression techniques can also be investigated for suitability of intended use [61]. These include mRNA Differential Display (DD), Representational Difference Analysis (RDA), Amplified Fragment Length Polymorphism (AFLP) and quantitative reverse transcriptase real time PCR (qRT-PCR).

Differential gene expression analysis was first performed using mRNA Differential Display (DD) [68]. During DD, cDNA is synthesized from mRNA of each sample of interest, followed by amplification using a combination of anchored oligo-dT and random oligonucleotides. The obtained differentially amplified fragments each represent a transcript or an expressed sequence tag (EST). The advantage of this technique is that it requires a small amount of bioinformatics application during data analysis. Improvements of the technique generated the second generation annealing control primer (ACP)-differential display RT-PCR [69]. Under optimal conditions of use, mRNA DD is a relatively inexpensive but powerful tool, used to identify and isolate differentially expressed transcripts, as well as for comparative studies between several mRNA populations [70].

Subtractive hybridization of mRNA is another method that has been employed to differentially identify mRNAs associated with a cell- or tissue type or cellular responses [71]. A reduction in the number of genes in need of analysis in a comparative transgenic study is an important advantage [72]. Another advantage of the technique is its ability to reveal lower abundance transcripts [73], but the technique is also time consuming and labor intensive.

Representational Difference Analysis (RDA) is a subtractive DNA enrichment technique designed to identify differences between two genomes without quantifying expression levels [74]. The technique was later modified by using cDNA as template to facilitate the detection of rare transcripts. cDNA-RDA utilizes subtractive DNA enrichment in association with PCR amplification, where two cDNA populations are hybridized to analyze genes that are differentially expressed under set and differing conditions [61]. The obtained difference products are sequenced and analyzed to determine the difference in gene expression levels between the two genomes. A noted disadvantage of this technique is the high levels of labor it requires.

Amplified Fragment Length Polymorphism (AFLP) is a PCR-based technique that has been widely used for its advantages since it utilizes PCR analysis on a small amount of DNA for the identification of various polymorphisms [61]. Several applications have been reported for AFLPs and these include identification of the relatedness of cultivars [56] and the relatedness between transgenic offspring and parental plants [61]. Moreover, the use of mRNA expression analysis through cDNA-AFLPs allows for the evaluation of a large pool of genes differentially expressed between the transgenic and the traditional counterpart. Since it affords the researcher the ability to target coding regions, it facilitates gene expression analysis that leads to the identification of genes involved in different biological processes [61, 75].

Once candidate genes have been identified, qRT-PCR is generally used for quantitative gene expression analysis [76]. This sensitive, highly specific and broad range technique offers researchers the ability to investigate rare transcripts, as well as to analyze multigene families. qRT-PCR is also the technique of choice to measure and quantify expression levels of the inserted transgene(s). However, researchers can only benefit from the effectiveness of this technique if proper internal controls are included. These controls, also known as reference genes, normalize the expression analysis, since they are consistently expressed in tissues of interest under varying experimental treatments [77].

11. Conclusion

Due to the non-selective nature of traditional methods of genetic modification, the possibility exists that endogenous genes and their functions will be disrupted through the random integration of the transgene into the plant genome. This phenomenon is linked to unintended effects of genetic modification. Gene expression analysis is thus a crucial part of investigations into the effect of transgene insertion on endogenous gene expression. An understanding of the dynamics of the various available techniques is thus important in selecting the most appropriate technique(s) for the realization of the set objectives. Each method described above has its advantages and limitations. Furthermore, the choice of technique would depend on whether prior knowledge of the host genome is available or not. Using more than one technique in complement would ensure optimum results for investigating comparative / differential gene expression analysis in transgenic crops.

Acknowledgements

This work was supported by the South African Agricultural Research Council (ARC), Department of Science and Technology (DST), National Research Foundation (NRF), Potato South Africa (PSA) and the University of Johannesburg, South Africa.

Conflict of interest

The authors declare no conflict of interest.

Notes

A related version of this chapter was available in electronic format to delegates of the GMASSURE (Assuring Agricultural and Food Safety of Genetically Modified Organisms in Southern Africa) science and technology program, organized by the African Centre for Gene Technologies (ACGT), Pretoria, South Africa, 2015–2017.

Author details

Lerato B.T. Matsaunyane[1,2] and Ian A. Dubery[2*]

*Address all correspondence to: idubery@uj.ac.za

1 Agricultural Research Council—Vegetable and Ornamental Plants, Pretoria, South Africa

2 Department of Biochemistry, University of Johannesburg, Johannesburg, South Africa

References

[1] ISAAA (International Service for the Acquisition of Agri-biotech Application). Agricultural Biotechnology (A lot more than just GM crops); 2010. www.isaaa.org/resources/publications/agricultural_biotechnology/download/default.asp

[2] Kuzma J, Kokotovich A. Renegotiating GM crop regulation. EMBO Reports. 2011;**12**:883-888

[3] Brookes G, Barfoot P. Economic impact of GM crops: The global income and production effects 1996-2012. GM Crops & Food: Biotechnology in Agriculture and the Food Chain. 2014;**5**:65-75

[4] Lusser M, Parisi C, Plan D, Rodríguez-Cerezo E. Deployment of new biotechnologies in plant breeding. Nature Biotechnology. 2012;**30**:231-239

[5] James C. Global Status of Commercialized Biotech/ GM Crops. International Service for the Acquisition of Agri-Biotech Applications (ISAAA) Brief 42; 2010. www.isaaa. org/resources/publications/briefs/42/default.asp, Ithaca, NY, USA

[6] Anthony VM, Ferroni M. Agricultural biotechnology and smallholder farmers in developing countries. Current Opinion in Biotechnology. 2012;**23**:278-285

[7] Malarkey T. Human health concerns with GM crops. Mutation Research. 2003;**544**:217-221

[8] Bakshi A. Potential adverse health effects of GM crops. Journal of Toxicology and Environmental Health Part B. 2003;**6**:211-225

[9] AgResearch. GMOs—the Disadvantages; 2001. Available on: http://www.agresearch.co.nz/scied/search/biotech/gene_gmocons.htm

[10] Ekici K, Sancak YC. A perspective on GM food crops. African Journal of Agricultural Research. 2011;**6**:1639-1642

[11] Hansen G, Wright MS. Recent advances in the transformation of plants. Trends in Plant Science. 1999;**4**:226-231

[12] Gelvin SB. The introduction and expression of transgenes in plants. Current Opinion in Biotechnology. 1998;**9**:227-232

[13] Haber JE. Recombination: A frank view of exchanges and vice versa. Current Opinion in Cell Biology. 2000;**12**:286-292

[14] Ohba T, Yioshioka Y, Machida C, Machida Y. DNA rearrangements associated with the integration of T-DNA in tobacco: An example of multiple duplications of DNA around the integration target. The Plant Journal. 1995;**7**:157-164

[15] Christou P. Strategies for variety-independent genetic transformation of important cereals, legumes and woody species utilizing particle bombardment. Euphytica. 1995;**85**: 13-27

[16] Morikawa H, Sakamoto A, Hokazono H, Irifune K, Takahashi M. Mechanism of transgene integration into a host genome by particle bombardment. Plant Biotechnology. 2002;**19**: 219-228

[17] Bode J, Benham C, Knopp A, Mielke C. Transcriptional augmentation: Modulation of gene expression by scaffold/matrix-attached regions (S/MAR elements). Critical Reviews in Eukaryotic Gene Expression. 2000;**10**:73-90

[18] Adem M, Beyene D, Feyissa T. Recent achievements obtained by chloroplast transformation. Plant Methods. 2017;**13**:30

[19] Paul JW, Qi Y. CRISPR/Cas9 for plant genome editing: Accomplishments, problems and prospects. Plant Cell Reports. 2016;**35**:1417-1427

[20] Cunningham FJ, Goh NS, Demirer GS, Matos JL, Landry MP. Nanoparticle-mediated delivery towards advancing plant genetic engineering. Trends in Biotechnology. 2018. DOI: 10.1016/j.tibtech.2018.03.009. in press

[21] Pawlowski WP, Somers DA. Transgene inheritance in plants genetically engineered by microprojectile bombardment. Molecular Biotechnology. 1996;**6**:17-30

[22] Koncz C, Nemeth K, Redei GP, Schell J. T-DNA insertional mutagenesis in Arabidopsis. Plant Molecular Biology. 1992;**20**:963-976

[23] Laufs P, Autran D, Traas J. A chromosomal paracentric inversion associated with T-DNA integration in Arabidopsis. The Plant Journal. 1999;**18**:131-139

[24] Fladung M. Gene stability in transgenic aspen (*Populus*) I. Flanking DNA sequences and T-DNA structure. Molecular and General Genetics. 1999;**260**:574-581

[25] Kumar S, Fladung M. Transgene repeats in aspen: Molecular characterisation suggests simultaneous integration of independent T-DNAs into receptive hotspots in the host genome. Molecular and General Genetics. 2000;**264**:20-28

[26] Kritzkova L, Hrouda M. Direct repeats of T-DNA integrated in tobacco chromosome: Characterization of junction regions. The Plant Journal. 1998;**16**:673-680

[27] Castle LA, Errampalli D, Atherton TL, Franzmann LH, Yoon ES, Meinke DW. Genetic and molecular characterization of embryonic mutants identified following seed transformation in Arabidopsis. Molecular and General Genetics. 1993;**241**:504-514

[28] Filipenko EA, Filipenko ML, Deineko EV, Shumnyi VK. Analysis of integration sites of T-DNA insertions in transgenic tobacco plants. Cytology and Genetics. 2007;**41**:199-203

[29] De Buck S, De Wilde C, van Montagu M, Depicker A. Molecular Breeding. 2000;**6**:459-468

[30] Kononov ME, Basuner B, Gelvin SB. Integration of T-DNA binary vector "backbone" sequences into tobacco genome: Evidence for multiple complex patterns of integration. The Plant Journal. 1997;**11**:945-957

[31] Lee M-K, Kim H-S, Kim S-H, Park Y-D. T-DNA integration patterns in transgenic tobacco plants. Journal of Plant Biology. 2004;**47**:179-186

[32] Cellini F, Chesson A, Colquhoun I, Constable A, Davies HV, Engel KH, et al. Unintended effects and their detection in GM crops. Food and Chemical Toxicology. 2004;**42**:1089-1125

[33] Thomas CM, Jones DA, English JJ, Carroll BJ, Bennetzen JL, Harrison K, et al. Analysis of the chromosomal distribution of transposon-carrying T-DNAs in tomato using the inverse polymerase chain reaction. Molecular and General Genetics. 1994;**242**:573-585

[34] Barakat A, Gallois P, Raynal M, Mestre-Ortega D, Sallaud C, Guiderdoni E, et al. The distribution of T-DNA in the genomes of transgenic Arabidopsis and rice. FEBS Letters. 2000;**471**:161-164

[35] Iglesias VA, Moscone EA, Papp I, Neuhuber F, Michalowski S, Phelan T, et al. Molecular and cytogenetic analyses of stably and unstably expressed transgene loci in tobacco. Plant Cell. 1997;**9**:1251-1264

[36] Pedersen C, Zimmy J, Becker D, Jahne-Gartner A, Lorz H. Localization of introduced genes on the chromosomes of transgenic barley, wheat, triticale by fluorescence in situ hybridization. Theoretical and Applied Genetics. 1997;**94**:749-757

[37] Svitashev S, Ananiev E, Pawlowski WP, Somers DA. Association of transgene integration sites with chromosome rearrangements in hexaploid oat. Theoretical and Applied Genetics. 2000;**100**:872-880

[38] Liu YG, Mitsukawa N, Oosumi T, Whittier RF. Efficient isolation and mapping of *Arabidopsis thaliana* T-DNA insert junctions by thermal asymmetric interlaced PCR. The Plant Journal. 1995;**8**:457-463

[39] Matzke AJM, Matzke MA. Position effects and epigenetic silencing of plant transgenes. Current Opinion in Plant Biology. 1998;**1**:142-148

[40] Salvo-Garrido H, Travella S, Bilham LJ, Harwood WA, Snape JW. The distribution of transgene insertion sites in barley determined by physical and genetic mapping. Genetics. 2004;**167**:1371-1379

[41] Ten Hoopen R, Montijn BM, Veuskens JT, Oud OJ, Nanninga N. The spatial localization of T-DNA insertions in petunia interphase nuclei: Consequences for chromosome organization and transgene insertion sites. Chromosome Research. 1999;**7**:611-623

[42] Kearney J. Food consumption trends and drivers. Philosophical Transactions Of The Royal Society B: Biological Sciences. 2010;**365**:2793-2807

[43] Plahuta P, Raspor P. Comparison of hazards: Current vs. GMO wine. Food Control. 2007; **18**:492-502

[44] Dibden J, Gibbs D, Cocklin C. Framing GM crops as a food security solution. Journal of Rural Studies. 2013;**29**:59-70

[45] Mayet M. African demand for Tiger Brands to go GM-Free; 2013. www.acbio.org.za

[46] Wilson AK, Latham JR, Steinbrecher RA. Transformation-induced mutations in transgenic plants: Analysis and biosafety implications. Biotechnology and Genetic Engineering Reviews. 2006;**23**:206-234

[47] König A, Cockburn A, Crecel RWR, Debruyne E, Grafstroem R, Hammerling U, et al. Assessment of the safety of food derived from GM crops. Food and Chemical Toxicology. 2004;**42**:1047-1088

[48] FAO (Food and Agriculture Organization of the United Nations). How to feed the world in 2050; 2009. www.fao.org/fileadmin/templates/wsfs/docs/expert_paper/ How_to_Feed_the_World_in_2050.pdf

[49] OECD (Organisation for Economic Co-ordination and Development). Safety Evaluation of Foods Derived by Modern Biotechnology: Concepts and Principles. Paris: Organisation for Economic Co-ordination and Development; 1993 http://www.oecd.org/pdf/M00033000/M00033002.pdf

[50] ICSU (International Council for Science). New Genetics, Food and Agriculture: Scientific Discoveries: Societal Dilemmas; 2003. http://www.icsu.org, http://www.icsu.org/2_resourcecentre/INIT_GMOrep_1.php4

[51] FAO (Food and Agriculture Organization of the United Nations). The State of Food and Agriculture 2003–2004: Agricultural Biotechnology: Meeting the Needs of the Poor. FAO; 2004. http://www.fao.org/docrep/006/Y5160E/Y5160E00.HTM

[52] Sanvido O, Romeis J, Bigler F. Ecological impacts of GM crops: Ten years of field research and commercial cultivation. Advances in Biochemical Engineering/Biotechnology. 2007; **107**:235-278

[53] Wetenschappelijk Instituut Volksgezondheid. Guidelines for Molecular Characterization of GM Higher Plants to be Placed on the Market, According to Annex III B of Directive 2001/ 18/EC. Final version: February 18, 2003 WIV/1520/ADS/06–1095 1–4. Afdeling Bioveiligheid en Biotechnologie

[54] Stein AJ, Rodriguez-Cerezo E. International trade and the global pipeline of new GM crops. Nature Biotechnology. 2010;**28**:23-25

[55] Gebhardt C, Ritter E, Barone A, Debener T, Walkemeier B, Schachtschabel U, et al. RFLP maps of potato and their alignment with the homologous tomato genome. Theoretical and Applied Genetics. 1991;**83**:49-57

[56] McGregor CE, Lambert CA, Greyling MM, Louw JH, Warnich L. A comparative assessment of DNA fingerprinting techniques (RAPD, ISSR, AFLP and SSR) in tetraploid potato (*Solanum tuberosum* L.) germplasm. Euphytica. 2000;**113**:135-144

[57] Coombs JJ, Frank LM, Douches DS. An applied fingerprinting system for cultivated potato using simple sequence repeats. American Journal of Potato Research. 2004;**81**:243-250

[58] Lightbourn GJ, Jelesko JG, Veilleux RE. Retrotransposon-based markers from potato monoploids used in somatic hybridization. Genome. 2007;**50**:492-501

[59] Nováková A, Šimáčková K, Bárta J, Čurn V. Potato variety identification by molecular markers based on retrotransposon analyses. Czech Journal of Genetics and Plant Breeding. 2009;**45**:1-10

[60] Pattanayak D, Chakrabarti SK, Naik PS. Genetic diversity of late blight resistant and susceptible Indian potato cultivars revealed by RAPD markers. Euphytica. 2002;**128**:183-189

[61] Matsaunyane LBT, Oelofse D, Dubery IA. Detection and molecular analysis of transformation-induced unintended effects in the genome of potato modified with the apple (*Malus domestica*) polygalacturonase inhibiting protein 1 (*pgip1*) gene. Potato Research. 2016;**59**:129-147

[62] Green CD, Simons JF, Taillon BE, Lewin DA. Open systems: Panoramic views of gene expression. Journal of Immunological Methods. 2001;**250**:67-79

[63] Velculescu VE, Zhang L, Vogelstein B, Kinzler KW. Serial analysis of gene expression. Science. 1995;**270**:484-487

[64] Zheng C, Choquer M, Zhang B, Ge H, Hu S, Ma H, Chen S. LongSAGE gene-expression profiling of *Botrytis cinerea* germination suppressed by resveratrol, the major grapevine phytoalexin. Fungal Biology. 2011;**115**:815-832

[65] Kehoe DM. DNA microarrays for studies of higher plants and other photosynthetic organisms. Trends in Plant Science. 1999;**4**:38-41

[66] Schena M, Shalon D, Davis RW, Brown PO. Quantitative monitoring of gene expression patterns with a complementary DNA microarray. Science. 1995;**270**:467-470

[67] Wang Z, Gerstein M, Snyder M. RNA-Seq: a revolutionary tool for transcriptomics. Nature Reviews Genetics. 2009;**10**:57-63

[68] Liang P, Pardee AB. Differential display of eukaryotic messenger RNA by means of the polymerase chain reaction. Science. 1992;**257**:967-971

[69] Sanabria NM, Dubery IA. Differential display profiling of the Nicotiana response to LPS reveals elements of plant basal resistance. Biochemical and Biophysical Research Communications. 2006;**344**:1001-1007

[70] Djami-Tchatchou AT, Maake MP, Piater LA, Dubery IA. Isonitrosoacetophenone drives transcriptional reprogramming in *Nicotiana tabacum* cells in support of defense. PlosOne. 2015;**10**(2):e0117377

[71] Wieland I, Bolge G, Asouline G, Wigler M. A method for difference cloning: Gene amplification following subtractive hybridisation. Proceedings of the National Academy of Sciences USA. 1990;**87**:2720-2724

[72] Hubank M, Schatz DG. Identifying differences in mRNA expression by representational difference analysis of cDNA. Nucleic Acids Research. 1994;**22**:5640-5648

[73] Guimaraes JM, Lee F, Zlotnik A, McClanahan T. Differential display by PCR: Novel findings and applications. Nucleic Acids Research. 1995;**23**:1832-1833

[74] Lisitsyn N, Wigler M. Cloning the differences between two complex genomes. Science. 1993;**259**:946-951

[75] Ritter E, Ruiz de Galarreta JI, van Eck HJ, Sánchez I. Construction of a potato transcriptome map based on the cDNA–AFLP technique. Theoretical and Applied Genetics. 2008;**116**: 1003-1013

[76] Bustin SA, Benes V, Nolan T, Pfaffl MW. Quantitative real-time RT-PCR: A perspective. Journal of Molecular Endocrinology. 2005;**34**:597-601

[77] Dombrowski JE, Martin RC. Evaluation of reference genes for quantitative RT-PCR in *Lolium temulentum* under abiotic stress. Plant Science. 2009;**176**:390-396